The Cath Lab
An Introduction

The Cath Lab
An Introduction

David L. Lubell, M.D.
Division of Cardiology
Mount Sinai Hospital
  Medical Center
Associate Professor of Medicine
Chicago Medical School
Chicago, Illinois

Lea & Febiger   Philadelphia
1990

Lea & Febiger
600 Washington Square
Philadelphia, PA 19106-4198
U.S.A.
(215) 922-1330

Lea & Febiger (UK) Ltd.
145a Croydon Road
Beckenham, Kent BR3 3RB
U.K.

Library of Congress Cataloging-in-Publication Data

Lubell, David L.
    The cath lab : an introduction / David L. Lubell.
      p.   cm.
    Includes index.
    ISBN 0-8121-1262-8
    1. Cardiac catheterization—Handbooks, manuals, etc. I. Title.
    [DNLM: 1. Heart Catheterization.   WG 141.5.C2 L928c]
RC683.5.C25L83   1990
617.4′120754—dc20
DNLM/DLC
for Library of Congress   89-12621
                                                        CIP

PRINTED IN THE UNITED STATES OF AMERICA

Print number: 5 4 3 2 1

This book is dedicated to my devoted wife Renée, who has encouraged me throughout my medical career. It is also dedicated to the many wonderful nurses and technicians who worked with me in the cardiac catheterization laboratory for more than 25 years. Helen Dougherty deserves special mention; she was devoted and intelligent, and she epitomized the finest tradition of nursing.

Foreword

Several excellent textbooks on cardiac catheterization and angiography are available for the established practitioner of invasive cardiology and for cardiovascular fellows in training. None has adequately addressed the needs of our all-important cardiac catheterization team, however. Their performance ultimately determines whether the catheterization procedure will be a comfortable, safe, and productive experience for our patients. No matter how competent the attending cardiologist is, he must rely upon nurses and technicians to assist him in implementing nearly every aspect of the catheterization procedure.

This comprehensive work reflects the author's extensive personal experience in invasive cardiology and cardiac catheterization laboratory supervision. As chief of the Division of Cardiology at Chicago's Mount Sinai Hospital and Medical Center, Dr. Lubell has developed an invasive cardiology team that reflects the high standards of training, compassion, and quality assurance emphasized in his writing.

Dr. Lubell's book addresses the needs of the entire cardiac catheterization team. The interesting, informative, and easily understood text will be greatly appreciated by nurses, physiologic and radiologic technicians, medical students, and representatives of the many manufacturers and suppliers of equipment used in today's cardiac catheterization laboratory.

JOSEPH V. MESSER, M.D.
Professor of Medicine
Rush Medical College
Chicago, Illinois

Preface

The idea for writing this book arose from the need to quickly train two new nurses for cath lab duties. I attempted to find basic reference sources for them and was surprised that little or no appropriate material was available. Many texts exist in the field of cardiac catheterization, but they are generally designed for physicians and trainees in cardiac catheterization. They do not fill the needs of a nurse or technician trying to obtain an overview of the nature and conduct of the procedure. Thus, the text will not dwell on details of the surgical technique of performing an arterial cutdown or discuss in depth the significance of a raised left ventricular end diastolic pressure. The focus will be more general and geared mainly to the catheterization nurse and x-ray or laboratory technician. Medical students should also find the text useful as an overview when they are assigned to a patient undergoing catheterization. Medical residents are another group who can make use of a generally descriptive rather than detailed text on the subject. Finally, physicians preparing for catheterization training may also find the text a useful introduction.

Topics include a brief history of cardiac catheterization, why the procedure is performed, the general medical nature of the information derived, the various forms the procedure may take, the equipment used (including the x-ray apparatus), and, most importantly, how we manage and monitor the patient during the procedure. The discussion will pertain to laboratories generally working with adult patients. For pediatric catheterization the principles are similar, but some details are naturally different, such as anesthesia and temperature control.*

Since my background is mainly in cardiology, the concepts discussed here will have a different and perhaps broader scope than if I were trained in radiology. However, radiologists and radiographic principles have contributed significantly to the development of catheterization; the sharp separation into an "x-ray" or "cath" approach is artificial and counterproductive.

I hope this book will be an easily read introduction and orientation to the way cardiac catheterizations are performed and how the catheterization laboratory is used to derive clinically important information about the cardiovascular system in as safe and humane a manner as possible.

Chicago, Illinois   DAVID L. LUBELL

---

*In the early development of cardiac catheterization, most laboratories handled both adult and pediatric patients. Presently, a pediatric cardiologist catheterizes children, and may work in a specially designed laboratory or a general catheterization laboratory.

Acknowledgments

I would like to thank the many individuals who helped and encouraged me in this endeavor. Drs. Maurice Schwartz, Joseph V. Messer, and Hymie Kavin read the manuscript and made valuable suggestions. The personnel of the cath lab, the cardiology fellows, and my associate Dr. Lalchand Goyal agreed that there was a need for the book, and that the manuscript, as it developed, was fulfilling its purpose.

I am also indebted to my father, Dr. Albert J. Lubell, and my sister, Mrs. Myra Humphry, who worked with me on style. Mr. Robert Markel suggested ways to make the text more lively.

I also appreciate the support given me for the past 10 years by Dr. Schwartz, Chairman of the Department of Medicine, and by Mt. Sinai Hospital Medical Center, Chicago.

Mrs. Sybil Waring, medical illustrator from the Department of Pathology, Michael Reese Hospital, Chicago, is greatly appreciated for her time and effort and for the quality of her work. Herb Comess did the photography. A special thanks is owed to Dr. Martin Swerdlow, Chairman of Pathology, for allowing them to work on this project.

Finally, I have the utmost gratitude for my secretary, Mrs. Patricia Houston, who typed and retyped the manuscript many times, always with good cheer.

Contents

The Cath Lab
An Introduction

1

History and Introduction

Cardiac or vascular catheters (long, thin, semiflexible tubes) have been inserted into the circulation of animals for physiologic experiments since the middle of the 19th century. The first recorded insertion of a catheter into a human heart was in 1929 by a German surgeon, Dr. Werner Forssmann. Against the wishes of his superior, but with the assistance of a nurse, he introduced a urologic catheter into his own arm vein and passed it centrally to the right atrium. He reported only a slight pressure sensation when the catheter passed through the axillary region. Dr. Forssmann then calmly walked to the x-ray department for a chest film to confirm the position of the catheter. Before he could actually have the film taken, it was necessary for him to kick a well-meaning person in the shins to prevent him from pulling the catheter out of the good doctor's arm. Forssmann was severely criticized for his "outrageous" action, and his bold step was unappreciated by the rigid local medical circles. His further attempts at research and development received only marginal support. Years later Forssmann was recognized as a pioneer and received a Nobel prize (1956).

Forssmann did manage to insert a catheter into the right atrium of one patient, who was dying of sepsis, for drug and fluid administration. The initial development of vascular catheterization, however, was in the direction of diagnosis, that is, pressure and flow measurements and angiography. More recently catheterization has been adopted for therapy, as illustrated by the techniques of intra-arterial or intra-coronary thrombolysis and angioplasty.

Following Forssmann's innovation, the intracardiac catheter was used sporadically until further investigation and development by Dr. André Cournand working at Bellevue Hospital in New York. Cournand and colleagues used the catheter to study the human circulation and, in particular, pulmonary physiology. Their work began before World War II and progressed steadily after the war. A large number of papers reported on patients with pulmonary emphysema and fibrosis.

1

Thereafter, much impetus for the development of cardiac catheterization came from pediatricians. As early as 1945, Brannon et al. described the diagnosis of atrial septal defect and Baldwin described the diagnosis of ventricular septal defect.

By today's standards the early x-ray techniques were primitive, angiographic contrast media (the so-called "dye") were not well tolerated, and dye injectors were cumbersome and unreliable. Despite the limitations, innovative and pioneering physicians such as Dr. Israel Steinberg, who worked at New York Hospital, were able to make an amazing array of diagnoses and advances. Most of this early work was accomplished from the venous side of the circulation.* An example of the limitation of the venous (right-heart) technique was its attempted use in the x-ray demonstration of left-heart chambers, the thoracic aorta, and arterial branches. This required large amounts of dye injected either into peripheral veins or the pulmonary artery with subsequent exposure of the x-ray films after the dye had traversed the pulmonary circulation. Useful in some, the results were often not diagnostic and were possibly harmful in others.

The development of left-heart and arterial catheterization was slower.** Simple arterial pressure recording and blood sampling techniques had been practiced by Cournand and others. An early technique for the x-ray demonstration of the abdominal aorta and peripheral arteries required the injection of dye through a needle inserted percutaneously into the lumbar region and advanced blindly into the aorta. H. Zimmerman (1950) showed that it was possible to pass a catheter from the brachial artery to the left ventricle.

Other early attempts at reaching the left circulation (which essentially are now only of historical interest) are puncture of the left atrium via the left main stem bronchus, paravertebral percutaneous puncture, and the supraclavicular "skewer" technique. Another percutaneous chest puncture technique that is still utilized on rare occasions is the direct apical left ventricular puncture, or parasternal left ventricular puncture.

These relatively primitive, not to say risky, means of catheterizing the left circulation have been mostly superceded by the retrograde brachial artery procedure developed by Dr. Mason Sones at the Cleveland Clinic (1962), and by percutaneous

---

*Catheterization of the veins is also known as "right-heart" catheterization, since by following the flow of blood in the veins (except in rare forms of congenital heart disease) the catheter reaches the right atrium, the right ventricle, etc.

**"Left-heart" or arterial catheterization is the term used for direct entry to the left-heart chambers with a needle or (more commonly) by reaching the heart by passing a catheter through an artery in the retrograde direction, that is, opposite the normal direction of blood flow.

retrograde puncture and catheterization of the femoral artery originated by Seldinger (1953) and further developed by Dr. Melvin Judkins, a radiologist. These techniques were utilized for selective coronary angiography, a major advance over the previous indirect or nonselective approaches. Finally, Ross and Brockenbrough at the National Institutes of Health, devised the transseptal puncture technique, whereby a needle/catheter enters the left atrium from the right atrium after puncture of the inter-atrial septum. These advances have resulted in the development of "modern" catheterization techniques. Today the Sones and Judkins techniques are the most commonly used and provide direct access to the left-heart structures, the coronary arteries, and most of the major peripheral arteries.

Finally, there is the development of interventional catheterization. Here the catheterization procedure is no longer limited to diagnosis but is used to perform a vascular or cardiac manipulation (i.e., "surgery") or to adminster medication (shades of Forssmann). Examples of interventional catheterization include the plugging of arteries supplying a site of internal hemorrhage (e.g., bleeding tumor), balloon angioplasty of a peripheral vessel or a coronary artery (Grünzig, 1979), and the infusion of streptokinase into a coronary artery obstructed by a thrombus as developed by Rentrop. Further discussion of some of these methods will appear in later chapters.

It should also be emphasized that the tremendous clinical interest in catheterization of the circulation stimulated the development of refined and innovative catheters (e.g., balloon-tipped catheters), improved angiographic dye, and remarkable advances in x-ray imaging equipment. The original laboratories and equipment were painfully primitive in comparison to their modern counterparts. The laboratories that we take for granted today are a result of the dedicated work of many physicians, nurses, technicians, and engineers.

SUMMARY

The history of the development of cardiovascular catheterization is fascinating, particularly for those who have had the opportunity to see it unfold before their eyes. However, more important to current day workers in the laboratory is that some understanding of the history and background of catheterization makes it clear that most "modern" procedure techniques have evolved from less precise or more cumbersome techniques. An example would be the development of selective angiography compared to the earlier nonselective (indirect) angiography.

2

The Catheterization Team

The proper performance and conduct of a cardiovascular procedure clearly requires a team approach. A complete list of catheterization laboratory personnel includes physician(s), nurses, x-ray technicians, darkroom technicians, laboratory technicians, and a receptionist/secretary. Not every laboratory uses such an extensive roster and in many laboratories people serve multiple functions. This chapter will describe the role and function of the various team members.

1. The *physician* actually performing the procedure and directing the team can be a cardiologist, radiologist, or pediatrician (less commonly a surgeon). Each physician will have been specifically trained in doing procedures and, in many laboratories, have had their credentials reviewed and approved. Performance may also be monitored (see chapter 16). In laboratories that participate in catheterization training programs, physician trainees (fellows) will perform phases of the catheterization procedures to a greater or lesser extent, depending on their level of experience, but always under the direct supervision of a trained cardiologist.

In preparing for a particular catheterization, the physicians should brief the team on the nature of the patient's problem and, as far as possible, on the "game plan" of the procedure. In this way the assistants are alerted to the specific needs of the case. For example, biopsy equipment may be needed. It may be necessary to request personnel from the pathology department to come to the laboratory and assist in the handling of specimens. Special catheterization table exercise equipment may have to be set up, or the respiratory therapy department may have to be notified to assist with a patient requiring mechanical ventilation. Biochemical testing of blood (lactate, renin) requires preparation of special reagents. All individuals participating and assisting with a procedure will function better when given the opportunity to prepare.

2. *Nurses* have traditionally been part of the team. Their background experience can be varied: critical care nurse, O.R.

nurse, nurse anesthetist. It takes a period of training, some 4 to 6 months (best under the guidance of an experienced cath lab nurse assisted by a physician) before a nurse can absorb the considerable amount of information and knowledge to function independently. On-the-job training is indispensable.

The most important function of the nurse is to prepare and monitor the patient. This includes observation of vital signs, such as respiration and blood pressure, and ECG monitor surveillance for evidence of arrhythmias. The subjective state of the patient must not be neglected either. In the semi-darkened catheterization laboratory, with the physician concentrating on a difficult catheterization manipulation, the nurse is a vital link between physician and patient. The physician will expect timely reports from the nurse as to the well-being of the patient and will want to be immediately informed of significant changes. From time to time the nurse will be directed by the physician to give various medications, such as nitroglycerine, atropine, and vasopressors. A working knowledge of the pharmacology of cardiovascular drugs is thus essential. Particularly in smaller laboratories, the nurse may function as the physician's surgical assistant, helping with cutdowns, compressing vessels, etc.

The nurse will become familiar with the conduct of the various types of procedures. For example, the instrument set-up for a pediatric case requiring the taking of many blood samples is quite different from the preparation for coronary angioplasty.

Finally, the nurse must become familiar with the wide variety of catheters, guidewires, sheaths, cutdown instruments, and other instruments. Basic understanding of the operating controls of the x-ray table, principles of radiation safety, and sterility practice is also required.

Parenthetically, it should be noted that the supply of catheterization laboratory nurses has recently become more limited, both because of the generally decreasing enrollment of nurse trainees and the creation of many new laboratories. Some laboratories with multiple catheterization facilities are trying to function without special catheterization nurses by using operating room nurses or nurse technicians instead. This is an expedient but unproven solution to the problem.

3. The *x-ray technicians* have previously received general training and are licensed. Those who work in a catheterization laboratory or angiography unit in a Department of Radiology are known as Special Procedure technicians. This means that they have been trained to operate the special catheterization x-ray equipment, which includes fluoroscopy, cine angiography, rapid film angiography, darkroom development of the exposed film, and darkroom quality control. In addition, many x-ray technicians are

able to operate the catheterization recording equipment. Depending upon circumstances in a particular laboratory, the x-ray technician may also perform other duties, such as setting up the catheterization equipment, preparing the patient for monitoring, and helping with ECG monitoring.

4. *Laboratory technicians* trained in general biochemical laboratory techniques are frequently employed in catheterization laboratories. Specifically, they take and analyze expired air samples for oxygen consumption, analyze blood samples for such properties as oxygen content and saturation, and calculate cardiac output. In some cases they perform biochemical analyses such as blood lactate determinations. Although modern technology has simplified some of the tests (e.g., direct reading oxygen saturation devices, or oximeters), many laboratories still rely on the "gold standard" Van Slyke method for blood gas content and Scholander microtechniques for air-sample analysis. Both of these techniques require considerable skill.

5. The *receptionist/secretary* position does not require specialized training but does require familiarity with catheterization laboratory scheduling. This person will often transcribe and prepare the catheterization reports from dictated tapes and maintain the record file. The secretary also monitors the myriad phone messages in and out of the laboratory and handles the frequent visitors, sales representatives, and other callers.

6. *Supervision and Interactions:* Most laboratories have a designated physician-director, usually an experienced individual knowledgeable in all aspects of laboratory function and management. The director has the overall responsibility for standards and practice and can assist all personnel in carrying out their functions.

In most laboratories a senior nurse or x-ray technician functions as a supervisor. This role includes personnel management such as work schedules and vacations, assessment of performance, and hiring and dismissals. Other important functions include ordering supplies and equipment, obtaining immediate service on malfunctioning equipment, and scheduling preventive maintenance service. The director works closely with the laboratory supervisor on all these matters.

It should be emphasized that the "job descriptions" of the various catheterization laboratory personnel positions are not rigid. A considerable degree of overlap exists and is desirable. Everyone working in the laboratory is part of a team. The team members support and help each other, remembering that the goal is to "produce" a catheterization procedure that is clinically useful, safe, and humane.

SUMMARY

This chapter sketches the "job descriptions" of the personnel who function in a modern catheterization laboratory. The roster varies from laboratory to laboratory and some individuals have overlapping areas of responsibility. In the subsequent chapters, as the technical aspects of the procedures are described, it should be possible to discern the roles of the different "team" members.

3

Indications for Cardiovascular Catheterization

Utilizing cardiovascular catheterization as a diagnostic test, we can answer specific clinical questions about the heart and circulation. For example, when coronary artery disease is clinically suspected, catheterization with the performance of coronary angiography can clinch the diagnosis. One can assess the degree of ventricular function impairment or the severity of pulmonary hypertension. Insofar as it is possible, a catheterization procedure is designed to have a clinical focus and is used to answer specific clinical questions. Such a procedure is not undertaken in the sense of an "exploration."

Since the introduction of catheterization into clinical practice there have been changes in the prevalence of certain cardiac diseases as well as marked technologic advances. The result has been a change in the clinical profile of patients undergoing catheterization. Coronary artery disease is the most common reason for catheterizing patients today. Previously, valvular heart disease was a much more frequent indication.

In addition to its clinical uses, cardiovascular catheterization is a powerful research tool without which many great medical advances would not have been possible. Coronary artery bypass operations, for example, were pioneered at the Cleveland Clinic as a direct result of Sones' development of selective coronary angiography. Detailed analysis and study of coronary circulation, normal and diseased, became possible in the living patient.

Another important way that catheterization is used in research is in the testing of cardiac drugs. For example, in patients with heart failure one can measure the effects of an experimental drug on pulmonary artery wedge pressure and cardiac output.

The following is a description of the main cardiovascular disease profiles in which cardiac catheterization can contribute important information to the clinical assessment.

8

CORONARY ARTERY DISEASE

Atherosclerotic plaque blockage of the (epicardial) coronary arteries leads to insufficient blood flow to the heart muscle. Patients with this disease often experience some form of angina or have sustained a myocardial infarction. In some instances, the patient may have congestive heart failure (without a clear-cut history of angina or infarction—so-called "ischemic" cardiomyopathy). When angina or infarction is the main problem, a "simple" left-heart catheterization can be performed.* This entails percutaneous retrograde arterial catheterization via the femoral artery or direct exposure of the brachial artery ("cut-down" technique) with the objective of obtaining a left ventriculogram and selective left- and right-coronary arteriograms.

When congestive failure has occurred as a result of coronary artery disease, either "silent" or overt, the cardiologist may also want to record right-heart pressures and determine cardiac output, and in this case, the right-heart catheterization is usually performed first. The pressure and flow determinations and angiographic appearance of the coronary arteries (stenotic, obstructed, etc.) and the left ventricle (dilated, areas of reduced or absent contraction, etc.) enable the cardiologist to assess the condition and plan management. For example, the results of the catheterization may help in deciding whether surgical or medical treatment is appropriate for a given patient.

A case in illustration was a 50-year-old woman, who was admitted to the CCU with symptoms and findings of congestive heart failure. We determined that the cause of this condition was a recently sustained, relatively small myocardial infarction. She responded initially to medical treatment, and further evaluation indicated that infarction had also occurred previously. A second episode of congestive heart failure then developed, which made us proceed promptly with catheterization. A "left-heart" procedure was undertaken and we found that the diastolic pressure was markedly elevated in the left ventricle and that overall ventricular function, assessed by left ventricular angiography, was reduced with a local area of noncontraction at the ventricular apex. The abnormal pressure and angiogram explained why the patient easily developed congestive failure. The underlying cause of the ventricular dysfunction was revealed by the coronary

---

* Actually, there is controversy over this point. Some cardiologists believe that "routine" right-heart catheterization is always required, even in cases of ordinary angina. I agree, however, with the position taken by the Society of Cardiac Angiography that routine right-heart catheterization is unnecessary unless there are specific complicating factors, such as heart failure.

angiograms, which showed severe stenosis of the proximal anterior descending branch and diagonal branch, as well as the circumflex branch.

Our assessment was that further medical treatment would not be effective. However, we had reservations about surgical revascularization by saphenous vein bypasses because of the possibility that damage to the myocardium (heart muscle) may have already been too extensive. By other means of testing we demonstrated a potential for improvement in myocardial function with revascularization. After coronary artery bypass grafting the patient experienced a remarkable clinical improvement and freedom from congestive failure. Echocardiography showed better ventricular function.

The catheterization procedure was a key element in the evaluation of this patient, allowing us to assess the coronary arteries for their suitability for bypass.

VALVULAR DISEASE

Patients with valvular disease continue to be seen in the United States, despite the marked decline in the prevalence of rheumatic heart disease.* In the past this was the most common cause of valvular disease, typically leading to mitral stenosis.

Other causes of valve disease include mitral valve prolapse (mitral insufficiency) and degenerative valve changes (aortic stenosis). There has been a dramatic increase in the incidence of bacterial endocarditis (mostly in I.V. drug abusers), which results in aortic, mitral, and tricuspid (rarely pulmonic) insufficiency, embolization, and congestive heart failure.

Manifestations of valvular stenosis or insufficiency include reduced activity and exercise capacity, congestive heart failure, syncope (in patients with aortic stenosis), arrhythmias, and systemic and pulmonary emboli. Patients with limiting symptoms, such as breathlessness with ordinary activity (N.Y. Heart Association Class III), would be considered candidates for catheterization. The procedure generally would include right-heart catheterization for cardiac output and right-heart and pulmonary capillary ("wedge") pressure determinations, and left-heart catheterization for left ventricular and aortic pressure determination. In addition, angiography of the left ventricle and coronary angiography is almost always included in these patients.

Such comprehensive testing is used to document valvular insufficiency and stenosis, rule out involvement of valves not

* In some parts of the world (e.g., India, China, and South Africa) rheumatic valvular disease remains common.

thought to be abnormal by other means, assess ventricular function, and determine the state of the coronary arteries, particularly in older patients. This information is crucial in helping to decide if a patient should undergo surgical valve repair or replacement.

To illustrate, a 33-year-old woman was admitted to the hospital with symptoms of mild to moderate congestive failure. Examination revealed mitral regurgitation, and initial medical management was successful. There was no evidence of infection (bacterial endocarditis) or coronary disease. We suspected mitral valve prolapse (MVP) with myxomatous degeneration of the mitral valve. Although MVP does not commonly cause congestive failure, the condition is serious when it does. Therefore, a right- and left-heart catheterization was undertaken. The right-heart data revealed a normal cardiac output and the absence of significant pulmonary hypertension. From the left-heart procedure we noted severe mitral regurgitation, good ventricular function, and normal coronary arteries. We recommended mitral valve surgery because the magnitude of the regurgitation in a patient who experienced congestive failure would eventually lead to irreversible ventricular dysfunction. At that time, valve repair would be no longer useful.

After some months delay, as the patient noted further reduction in exercise capacity, the mitral valve was replaced, restoring the patient to normal function. She was still well 3 years later. The catheterization procedure pinpointed the diagnosis and gave us the confidence to make a rational recommendation.

CONGESTIVE HEART FAILURE AND CARDIOMYOPATHY

Patients may develop congestive heart failure from a variety of causes, including coronary and valve disease, as mentioned above, and congenital heart disease. The term "cardiomyopathy" is used when a disease process affects the heart muscle (myocardium) directly, resulting in depressed pump function, most often with dilated cardiac chambers (dilated cardiomyopathy). Etiologies are diverse and include chronic alcoholism, viral myocarditis, and drug toxicity (anticancer drugs such as doxorubicin). Heart muscle may also be infiltrated with amyloid (a proteinaceous fibrillar material) or sarcoid (inflammatory) granuloma.

These patients undergo catheterization to determine cardiac output and assess the degree of ventricular dysfunction and hemodynamic abnormalities. Coronary angiography is performed to rule out coronary disease.

Such patients may also be candidates for endomyocardial biopsy, which can be diagnostic in conditions such as cardiac amyloid or myocarditis. The cause of the patient's cardiomyopathy, however, often remains unexplained.

Cor pulmonale, which literally means heart disease caused by lung disease, is another form of heart disease that can appear clinically as congestive failure. A disease process that results in pulmonary parenchymal destruction and pulmonary vascular obstruction raises the resistance to blood flow and pressure in the pulmonary circuit (pulmonary hypertension), which increases the work of the right ventricle. Eventually, right ventricular pumping function becomes depressed and clinical "right" heart failure develops (engorged neck veins and liver, edema, sometimes ascites, etc.).

Pulmonary diseases that can cause cor pulmonale include fibrosis, bullous emphysema, cystic fibrosis, recurrent pulmonary emboli, far-advanced tuberculosis, parasitic disease, pneumoconiosis, and pulmonary vascular obstruction without demonstrable cause (primary pulmonary hypertension).

A right-heart catheterization in cor pulmonale shows very high pulmonary artery pressure (90 to 100 mm systolic in severe cases) and vascular resistance with normal or only mildly increased "wedge" pressure (i.e., the pulmonary hypertension is not caused by left-heart failure). Cardiac output is decreased in later stages of the disease.

CONGENITAL HEART DISEASE

Pediatric cardiologists usually catheterize infants and young children with congenital heart disease; adult cardiologists manage patients above 16 years old. Newborns or patients in early childhood with congenital heart disease present with cyanosis (right-to-left shunting through intracardiac defects), or they may have congestive failure. The latter can be caused by left-to-right intracardiac shunting, resulting in overperfusion of the lungs or obstructive lesions (e.g., pulmonic or aortic stenosis). Catheterization is usually performed in such cases for precise diagnosis and to assess severity. The procedure includes pressure measurements, shunt detection, and selective angiography. Palliative and, at times, curative surgical treatment may be undertaken, based on the findings.

During the procedure infants and small children obviously need careful sedation (in some cases general anesthesia), restraint, and maintenance of body warmth. The procedure is most often carried out by cutdown in the subinguinal area over the femoral vein and artery or saphenous vein (in older children). Congenital heart disease can go undetected until adulthood.

Some time ago, a 25-year-old man came to our clinic, referred for the assessment of a murmur. He had a history of hypertension and complained of headaches and sexual dysfunction. Femoral pulses were absent and diffuse bruits could be auscultated in the neck and behind the left shoulder. There was also telltale rib-notching noted on the chest x ray. The clinical diagnosis was coarctation of the aorta.

An aortic angiogram obtained after passage of a catheter from the right brachial artery, retrograde to the aortic root, showed a classic symmetric narrowing of the aorta just distal to the left subclavian artery (which supplied a huge collateral circulation) and a bulbous dilation of the aorta just below the narrowed segment.

After surgical correction of the lesion, the blood pressure slowly normalized and sexual dysfunction was no longer present. (The latter was caused by the low arterial pressure in the aorta below the coarctation.) Thus the catheterization procedure (essentially an aortic angiogram in this case) confirmed the clinical diagnosis and pointed the way for definitive treatment.

EMERGENCY PROCEDURES

Two procedures are commonly performed on an emergency basis. The first is pulmonary angiography (basically a right-heart catheterization) when pulmonary embolism is suspected. The second is aortography in cases of suspected dissecting hematoma of the aorta or aortic rupture after chest trauma. Gunshot wounds to the chest and chest trauma (steering wheel injury) can also be a reason for an emergency procedure.

Other conditions for which emergency catheterization may be required are complications of acute myocardial infarction (e.g., rupture of the intraventricular septum or papillary muscle with mitral regurgitation) or infectious endocarditis with acute valvular insufficiency. (Thrombolytic therapy and coronary angioplasty in acute myocardial infarction will be discussed in chapters 13 and 14.)

An example of an emergency catheterization was the case of a 17-year-old woman accidentally shot in the chest. Aside from agitation on initial examination, symptoms were minimal. A small entrance wound was present anteriorly. No obvious exit wound was found. The chest x ray showed slight widening of the mediastinum and no sign of the bullet. A pulmonary angiogram was recommended by the surgeon, but as we prepared to do this, the patient's condition deteriorated. A systolic/diastolic murmur developed, suggesting an arteriovenous connection; we elected to obtain an aortogram instead. By the time the patient was placed on the procedure table, intubation for pulmonary edema was required. We started by scanning the body with the fluoróscope and located the bullet in the right leg just below the inguinal ligament. The aortic root angiogram was accomplished by retrograde arterial catheterization from the left groin (femoral artery). Contrast media freely entered the left ventricle from the aorta (massive aortic regurgitation) and also opacified the left atrium. The patient was quickly taken to surgery. The surgeon found that the bullet had entered the right ventricle anteriorly, pierced the upper part of the interventricular septum, tore the root of the aorta, therby causing aortic valve regurgitation, and then passed through the posterior wall of the aorta, entering the left atrium. Since the bullet was later found in the right superficial artery, we concluded that it had migrated into the left ventricle and had been carried by the blood to the leg (embolization). Miraculously, no major coronary branch was injured. The surgeon heroically repaired the rent in the back wall of the aorta, replaced the damaged aortic valve, repaired the septum, closed the hole in the right ventricle, and removed the bullet and repaired the femoral artery. The patient recovered completely and was "normal" except for the presence of the prosthetic aortic valve.

The results of the emergency angiogram enabled the surgeon to undertake life-saving surgery.

PERIPHERAL ANGIOGRAPHY

Arterial insufficiency, usually of the lower extremities, is a common problem occurring mainly in older patients. It is generally a result of atherosclerotic narrowing of the arterial tree, which often begins in the lower aorta and involves any site below. Diabetes mellitus, hypertension, smoking, and elevated serum cholesterol contribute to the development of the disease. The usual symptoms are exercise-induced (ischemic) pain in the hip, thigh, or calf (intermittent claudication) or, in severe cases, rest pain and tissue breakdown (gangrene).

Angiographic demonstration of the lower body circulation (e.g., location of obstructions and collateral formation) is often useful in planning treatment. Retrograde percutaneous catheterization via the femoral artery can be performed in most instances. When that procedure is not possible, the brachial artery technique can be used.

Peripheral angiography (including imaging of the visceral branches of the aorta and cerebral angiography) is frequently performed in the radiology department. Cardiologists can also be involved in this type of work, particularly when brachial arterial cutdowns are required.

ARRHYTHMIA

Some patients are subject to debilitating or life-threatening cardiac rhythm disturbances for which analysis of the electrophysiologic events, as detected directly in the heart ("internal" electrocardiogram), can be of use. This is known as electrophysiologic studies (EPS). Arrhythmia may be a manifestation of coronary artery disease, valvular disease, cardiomyopathy, and even congenital heart disease.

For example, after a myocardial infarction (particularly a large one with left ventricular aneurysm formation) there may be frequent premature ventricle beats and short or long runs of ventricular tachycardia or ventricular fibrillation. The latter two abnormal rhythms can be fatal and require an attempt at prevention. Traditionally, the therapy is a more or less trial-and-error testing of the clinical efficacy of a variety of antiarrhythmic drugs.

By inserting one or more bipolar or multipolar electrode catheters into the heart (usually the right heart by the intravenous route), it is possible to obtain information such as atrium-to-His bundle conduction time, His bundle to ventricular conduction time, and right-to-left atrium conduction time. The electrodes can also be used for electrical stimulation of the atrium, the ventricle, and even the His bundle.

In the case of the postinfarction patient with serious ventricular arrhythmia, it may be useful to electrically stimulate the right ventricle in an attempt to induce tachycardia. The patient can then be treated, while on the catheterization table, with a series of antiarrhythmic drugs in an attempt to find one or a combination that is most effective at inhibiting the induction of tachycardia or at preventing induction completely. The expectation is that the selected drug, administered chronically, will be effective in reducing the severity of spontaneous arrhythmia or preventing it altogether.

CONTRAINDICATIONS FOR CATHETERIZATION

We have reviewed the main reasons why patients undergo catheterization and angiography. There are also clinical situations in which catheterization is ill-advised or the risk excessively outweighs the benefit. This applies to elective procedures usually undertaken for diagnosis and to formulate treatment plans. As mentioned above, emergency procedures may be required in patients who may be desperately ill (e.g., pulmonary angiography in suspected pulmonary emboli or coronary angioplasty (PTCA) in acute myocardial infarction with shock).

Acute clinical conditions that are considered contraindications to elective catheterization procedures include: fever and infection (septic state), anemia, hemorrhage, bleeding tendency (e.g., low platelet count), shock, hypoxia, electrolyte imbalance, uncontrolled hypertension, arrhythmia, decompensated congestive heart failure, and acute myocardial infarction. Patients may be able to undergo catheterization after correction or treatment of these conditions.

We also avoid elective procedures in patients with chronic end-stage disease such as cancer or dementia. There may be technical reasons, such as difficult vascular access or body or limb deformities, that could make catheterization inappropriate.

SUMMARY

We have reviewed the utilization of cardiac catheterization as a diagnostic test and as a research tool. The majority of patients requiring catheterization today have potential or actual coronary artery disease, in contradistinction to the early period of catheterization when valvular and congenital disease was more common. The case illustrations point out the central importance of catheterization data in evaluating patients for cardiac surgical treatment. Contraindications for catheterization are also discussed.

4

Preparing for the Procedure and Monitoring the Patient

It is the responsibility of the physician or cardiologist to inform the patient about the reasons for undergoing catheterization. The American Heart Association publishes a booklet that is useful in helping patients learn about and understand the procedure.

Precatheterization testing, which the patient can have on an outpatient basis a few days before the procedure, includes a 12-lead ECG, a chest x ray (if a recent one is not available), a CBC, and measurements of BUN creatinine, electrolytes, pro-thrombin time (PT), partial thrombo-plastin time (PTT), and possibly blood glucose. The prothrombin time should definitely be less than 18 seconds, preferably less than 15 sec.

In some hospitals members of the catheterization team, in particular the nurse, participate with the cardiologist (who is ultimately responsible) in obtaining the patient's informed written consent before the procedure. A frank (but not necessarily graphic) description of the procedure, including how it will be done (e.g., brachial or femoral approach) and its main risks, should be given to virtually all patients. Although, strictly speaking, cardiovascular catheterization is a surgical operation, albeit perhaps a "mini" operation, we present it to the patient as a test (exception: interventional catheterization procedures; see chapters 13 and 14).

A brief description of the laboratory is appropriate. On occasion, some individuals express a desire, which should be honored, to view the laboratory beforehand. Most patients will also appreciate knowing, for example, that they will not be given general anesthesia, but will receive sedation and local anesthesia ("as a dentist does to pull a tooth"), that they will be able to communicate with the nurse and doctor and ask questions, and that they will be requested to perform certain breathing maneuvers. Expressions like "we will shoot dye" should be avoided, as such words can be misunderstood. A substitute would be "we will inject liquids that we can see on x ray." During the discussion, it

17

is imperative to ask the patient about drug allergies and if there has been a prior angiographic dye reaction. The latter does not automatically preclude angiography but may necessitate pretreatment with corticosteroids and antihistamine. The newer, allegedly less allergenic contrast media can also be used.

In cases in which there is a language barrier and no one from the catherization team can communicate with the patient, it is desirable to find someone (even a member of the patient's family) to assist during the procedure as translator. It is imperative that a patient be able to express, for example, that he or she is experiencing chest pain.

When the procedure is scheduled for the morning, the patient is maintained in a fasting state during the preceding night. However, important oral medications, such as beta blockers or digitalis, can be given in a sip of water an hour before the catheterization. For procedures at midday or in the afternoon the patient can safely be allowed a light breakfast, including liquids and toast, between 7 and 8 A.M. Lunch is omitted. When the patient is an insulin-dependent diabetic, only half of the usual morning dose of insulin is given. The physician is responsible for entering precatheterization orders into the patient's chart.

Before leaving the hospital room (or upon arrival in the catheterization laboratory in the case of an outpatient), the patient should be requested to empty his or her bladder. If necessary, the patient should use a urinal or bedpan before being wheeled into the catheterization room.

An intravenous line should be inserted either before the patient leaves the hospital room or in the preparation room, or anteroom, of the catheterization laboratory. This line should be an indwelling plastic cannula and must flow reliably, as it will be used for the administration of important medications.

Precatheterization sedation should be given when the catheterization laboratory calls the hospital unit for the patient. It can also be given to an outpatient upon arrival in the laboratory. Ordinarily this consists of 5 to 10 mg of diazepam (Valium) or 50 mg of hydroxyzine (Vistaril) in a few sips of water. In very anxious patients, meperidine (Demerol) (25 to 75 mg I.M.) can be used.

Before the patient enters the laboratory, the nurse will turn on and check the defibrillator, apply conductive paste to the electrode paddles,* and check the supply of emergency and other drugs. The cath lab room should be clean (with blood stains from previous cases removed from the floor by housekeeping, if necessary). Fresh linen is placed on the cleaned catheterization table.

---

*The nurse (and technicians) are expected to be familiar with the operation of the defibrillator.

It is convenient at this time to position the patient's x-ray identification plate (made up with lead characters) on the table and expose a short run of film for identification purposes. This can be done by the nurse or x-ray technician. It appears like this:

```
DOE, JOHN
Today's date
Cath # (or hosp. #)
Name of Hospital
```

This also ascertains that the machinery is ready to operate and that cine film is properly loaded.

The sterile instrument table should be set up according to the type of procedure planned. The nurse or technician prepares a variety of catheters and other equipment that may be used. Medications (lidocaine, heparin, etc.) and flush solutions are placed in appropriate containers (see chapter 15).

The patient is usually brought to the preparation room by Central Transport on a gurney. The patient is greeted and the chart reviewed for properly signed informed consent, administration of pre-cath medications, and recent blood tests (e.g., recent ECG, prothrombin time, CBC, BUN, creatinine). Abnormalities or changes should be brought to the physician's attention. This is the time to initiate the use of the catheterization procedure flow sheet. The form used in the Mount Sinai Hospital Medical Center, Chicago, laboratory is shown in chapter 15, but any similar form that permits sequential recording of the data can be used.

In some hospitals, the pubic hair shaving for groin procedures is done in the patient's room, but the cath lab personnel may be required to do this. Additional shaving of hair around the upper thigh makes it easier to remove the pressure bandage applied at the termination of a femoral procedure. Eyeglasses should be removed and carefully laid aside. Dentures should be taken out unless the patient needs them to hold a mouthpiece for expired air collection. (They should be removed thereafter.) The skin is prepared and ECG monitoring electrodes are put in place. Meticulous electrode placement is important because a good quality signal is needed throughout the procedure. Electrodes are firmly taped to the skin. Radiolucent electrodes and cables have recently become available and can be placed more centrally on the arm and chest without casting unwanted x-ray shadows. Also, by mounting these electrodes closer to the torso, arm movement (e.g., when the patient is requested to place the arms above the head during coronary angiography) causes less ECG signal artifacts.

Blood pressure and pulse are determined and recorded on the flow sheet. The patient is examined for signs of dyspnea and orthopnea. If the latter is present, the patient may not be able to lie comfortably on the cath table. For a femoral artery procedure, the dorsal pedal and posterior tibial pulses should be marked with a felt pen (both feet). The radial and ulnar pulses should be marked for a brachial artery procedure.

It is important to practice breath-holding and coughing with the patient. The patient will be asked to take and hold a deep breath for about 10 sec. during certain angiograms (coronary, ventricular, pulmonary). This causes the diaphragm to descend away from the heart region and increases x-ray contrast between the heart and lungs. Prompt, hard, repeated coughs are requested when coronary angiography produces excessive bradycardia. The patient can also be shown how to hold a mouthpiece for expired air collection, should this be planned.

The patient is now wheeled into the laboratory to a position alongside the catheterization table and can, with help, transfer him- or herself over. It is important to protect the patient from injury that might be caused by contact with surrounding machinery. When individuals are unable to make the transfer themselves, at least four people lift the sheet under the patient and use it as a sling to shift him or her onto the catheterization table. If necessary the patient can be slightly propped up by pillows under the back and head. It is important to keep the patient from chill by covering him or her with appropriate sheets or blankets.

The ECG leads are then attached and taped in place and the monitored ECG observed for trace stability as the leads are manipulated. It is also necessary to adjust the strain gauge, which is mounted on a movable bracket on the edge of the catheterization table, up or down so that it is positioned at the midchest level.

At this time one can review the instructions for breathing and coughing with the patient and also have the patient practice different positions on the table (e.g., half right or left turn) that may be used later during angiography.

On rare occasions it is necessary to perform catheterization in a patient who is comatose or requires a mechanical ventilator. It is imperative to have the respiratory technician in the procedure room to operate the ventilator and manage respiration. Also, if the possibility of a ventilatory arrest is anticipated, the anesthesiologist should be available in the laboratory. (A cath lab nurse or other personnel can perform emergency intubation if they are trained.)

The physician, nurse, or technician can then begin the cleansing and draping of the anatomical site to be used. Strain gauge tubing, manifolds, and flush and dye solutions are assembled; the procedure is ready to begin.

The nurses, technicians, and assistants have several important direct patient responsibilities during the course of the procedure. First and foremost, the essential responsibility for all individuals participating in the procedure is to maintain a constant awareness of the condition of the patient. Everyone must watch the ECG monitor and everyone—especially the nurse—must observe the patient for signs of alertness, comfort, pain, etc. This is made somewhat difficult by the dimmed lighting in the room during fluoroscopy and angiography. Pressure waveforms displayed on the monitor also need to be observed (hypertension or hypotension, damping, etc.). Any alterations that occur, such as rapid or slow ECG heart rates, frequent PVCs, pressure changes, or patient symptoms, must be brought to the attention of the cardiologist. Rhythm disturbances are most prone to occur when a catheter is positioned in the ventricle (left or right) during ventriculography and during coronary angiography. The experienced physician will have developed a strong sense of awareness of the patient's condition but must be able to rely on the assistants for additional information.

In the event of ventricular fibrillation (fortunately rare), the nurse or assistant will charge the defibrillator, apply the paddles, and discharge the shock at the physician's direction. Other forms of resuscitation may be required and all personnel must be instantly ready to assist with such measures as CPR, Ambu bag ventilation, and intubation (if trained).

The next important task is to maintain a careful flow-sheet record of the procedure, including the timing of incisions or punctures, what catheters are used, time of pressure recordings at particular sites, site of origin and time of blood samples, time of angiograms in a particular chamber, and the time, dose, and route of administration of the medication. Enter patient reactions and condition also.

It is often necessary to assist the physician and hand him or her a wide variety of instruments and equipment such as guidewires, catheters, and tubing. These are packaged in such a way that the external wrapping can be peeled back, allowing the operator to remove an inner sterile package with the desired item. The physician may also request that the nurse give various medications I.V. or orally at different times during the procedure. These medications can include I.V. atropine, sublingual nitroglycerine or nifedipine, I.V. nitroglycerine, antiarrhythmics, and pressor agents. Some medications are administered via a catheter by the physician. The administration of all medications must be documented in the flow-sheet record.

When an angiogram is about to be obtained (i.e., dye or contrast medium is about to be injected), it is important to warn the patient that he or she may experience a sense of heat or flushing, which ordinarily dissipates in a few seconds. Also, warn the patient that the camera(s) or film changer(s) make a lot of noise. The patient can be reminded to follow breathing instructions.

At the end of the procedure, once arm or groin bandages are in place, the nurse makes a final check of the blood pressures and pulse and observes the clinical state of the patient (breathlessness, chest pain, urticaria, etc.). The patient is assisted from the cath table to the gurney. The patient must not flex the hip on the side where a femoral procedure was performed or flex the arm after a brachial artery procedure. Manual pressure at the femoral site during the strain of moving helps maintain hemostasis. After being wheeled from the catheterization laboratory, the patient should be periodically observed for 10 or 15 min. while waiting in the recovery area for Central Transport to arrive.

Unless the cardiologist directs otherwise, the patient can be given oral liquids such as fruit juice or water and encouraged to drink freely. Once again the patient should be reminded not to bend the leg on the side of a femoral procedure or markedly flex the elbow after a brachial artery procedure for 4 hours. The patient should remain at bed rest for 4 to 6 hours after a femoral procedure but can ambulate after a brachial procedure when fully alert and stable.

The nurse or technician should then call the nursing unit to which the patient is to return and give a brief report of the procedure, any complications, and the blood pressure and pulse.

Finally, the catheterization flow-sheet record should be completed and the catheterization room prepared for the next patient.

In our laboratory, before the patient leaves the laboratory the cardiologist must enter a progress note in the patient's hospital chart as to what procedure was performed, any complications, and preliminary findings, if possible.

"OUTPATIENT" PROCEDURES

Some procedures can now be appropriately performed in outpatients. This undoubtedly has come about because the skills of the "team" have improved and because the equipment is superior (better x-ray imaging, use of sheaths, safer contrast media for angiograms, etc.). We also have the ability to screen patients better by using other noninvasive techniques.

Acceptable for outpatient procedures would be "low-risk" individuals without the following medical problems: unstable angina, congestive failure, aortic stenosis, and significant arrhythmias. Patients with uncomplicated stable angina requiring coronary angiography, or patients with peripheral vascular disease requiring aortography, are examples of those given consideration.

Preliminary testing, consent and instructions to the patient should be completed 1 or 2 days before the procedure. Outpatients are requested to come to the hospital early in the morning, when an ECG is recorded. The catheterization is performed in the early part of the day so that the patient can be observed for such conditions as delayed contrast medium reactions, bleeding, and arrhythmias for 3 to 6 hours before release, always accompanied by a relative or friend.

Outpatient procedures may prove to be an effective cost-saving measure, but for some patients it will represent a hardship. Consider the patient with angina (even if "stable") who has to travel 1 or 2 hours on a cold winter morning to arrive at the hospital at 7 or 8 A.M. A small but definite increase in morbidity (bleeding) also seems inevitable.

SUMMARY

This chapter provides a general description of what we do to prepare the patient for catheterization, how we observe and monitor the patient during the procedure, and what we need to do in the immediate postcatheterization period. The main points considered were: informing the patient about the nature of the procedure and informed consent, precatheterization laboratory testing, preparation of the catheterization laboratory, hookup of the ECG monitoring system, general instructions to the patient, making the patient comfortable on the table, constant surveillance of the patient and monitors (ECG, pressure wave forms) during the procedure, maintenance of the procedure record ("flow sheet"), administration of medication, obtaining and maintaining hemostasis after catheter removal, and discharging the patient from the laboratory.

5

Cardiac Catheterization: General Procedure

In this chapter we will review, in a general way, how we perform a cardiovascular catheterization. It is possible to catheterize patients of any age, from neonates to the aged. Advances in techniques and technology have made procedures faster and safer, broadening the indications for catheterization. Useful information can now be obtained in sicker patients. The management and techniques utilized for each patient should be preplanned and individualized. A "cookbook approach" is inappropriate because every patient manifests medical problems in a unique way.

Four kinds of information are derived from catheterization: vascular and cardiac pressure measurements; blood-flow determinations (e.g., cardiac output and shunt flows); angiography, which is an anatomic/functional "visualization," or imaging, of cardiac or vascular structures; and electrophysiologic studies.

Additional diagnostic information can be derived from the removal of tissue (biopsy) and biochemical testing of either blood samples taken from particular sites in the circulation. Renin concentrations in renal vein blood are useful in testing a patient for unilateral renovascular hypertension. Similarly, catecholamine concentrations in blood withdrawn from different locations in the inferior vena cava can help in locating a pheochromocytoma.

The procedure is performed with the patient resting on a catheterization table (or angiography table when performed in the Radiology Department). Basically, this is a radiolucent, padded operating table that allows physical access to the arm, groin, or occasionally the neck region. Also incorporated is x-ray machinery that permits radiographic monitoring of the position of the catheter in the circulatory system (fluoroscopy) and the visualization of injected angiographic dyes.

Electrocardiographic monitoring is mandatory in the catheterization laboratory, but is not routinely utilized in the radiology laboratory. All personnel directly involved with the procedure have the responsibility of observing the electrocardiograph mon-

24

itor for arrhythmia. Nurses or other laboratory personnel are also expected to observe the patient's vital signs and level of comfort, and to look for dye and drug reactions and other significant changes. Either before arriving at the catheterization laboratory or in the preparation room, the patient will receive some form of sedation. This may take the form of a sedative "cocktail" injected intramuscularly in infants or a small dose of tranquilizer or possibly a parenteral narcotic such as meperidine in an adult. Parenthetically, it may be mentioned that in the past, prophylactic antibiotics were commonly administered before the procedure. This practice is now no longer recommended.

Cardiovascular catheterization is carried out using sterile surgical technique. Individuals performing the procedure are expected to wear surgical scrub suits, caps, masks, and booties. At this point it is necessary for the operators to put on lead aprons and affix the radiation safety badges (see chapter 8). (The weight of the lead aprons is, in part, responsible for the fatigue experienced by those working in the catheterization room.)

Next, the operators perform a surgical scrub and then don sterile gowns and surgical gloves. Although sterile technique varies from laboratory to laboratory, we require that those individuals not directly participating in the procedure, but who may need to enter the laboratory, also wear scrub suits and masks.

After the catheterization site has been selected, the assistant or physician will prepare the site in the usual manner for surgical sterility. Povidone-iodine solution is commonly used. Sterile toweling or sheeting is used to isolate the area. When the groin area is utilized, the nearby pubic hair has been previously removed with a safety razor.

Sterile procedure and precautions protect both the patient and the operators. The incidence of wound infection or sepsis after catheterization is very low, approaching 0%.

The next step is to inject local anesthetic (usually lidocaine) into the skin and subcutaneous tissue over the vein or artery to be exposed by cutdown or punctured percutaneously. This may be somewhat painful for the patient, but in skilled hands the duration of the pain is brief and little further local discomfort persists during the procedure. During this injection some patients benefit from holding someone's hand and from gentle reassurance.

The operator then inserts a catheter into the vein or artery or both (see chapter 7 for insertion techniques). As the catheter is advanced centrally, the fluoroscope is activated so that the operator can observe its progress and manipulate it appropriately. The patient generally has little or no sensation of catheter movement since the catheter is, of course, moving in natural channels. Some discomfort is experienced as the catheter lodges against the wall of a vessel at a point of curvature. The operator is trained to gently withdraw, rotate, and advance the catheter as it is visualized fluoroscopically, until it reaches the desired position.

The external end of the catheter can be connected to a pressure-measuring apparatus. This consists of a stopcock arrangement and flexible tubing connected to a strain gauge, a device that converts the pressure waves into an electronic signal for display on a monitor. The waveform assists in determining the position of the catheter tip (e.g., in a ventricle). The desired waveforms are also available for permanent recording and analysis. In some procedures (particularly in pediatric catheterization) blood is withdrawn into heparinized syringes from the external end of the catheter with the tip at various sites within the circulatory system. Oxygen saturation determinations are then made which can be used to establish the presence or absence of intracardiac shunting. In the case of a ventricular septal defect, the oxygen saturation would be increased in blood sampled from the right ventricle and pulmonary artery, in comparison to samples taken from the right atrium and vena cavae.

Cardiac output is also commonly determined in the catheterization laboratory and is usually obtained in one of three ways. The oldest technique, commonly referred to as the "Fick," requires blood sampling from the pulmonary artery and a peripheral artery for oxygen content determination while oxygen consumption is determined by analyzing expired air collected in some form of tank or bag. The other techniques are modifications of the so-called Fick technique. The "dye" (or "indicator") dilution cardiac output is obtained by injecting indocyanine green into the pulmonary artery and "sampling" in a peripheral artery. A photometric device detects the appearance of the indicator as it circulates from the lung to the arterial circulation. The concentration buildup and subsequent "washout" depend on cardiac output.

Nowadays, using the Swan-Ganz catheter, thermal dilution output, with "cold" as the indicator, can be obtained by injecting cold solutions of known temperature into the right atrium and observing the thermal effects on the blood with the thermister mounted at the catheter tip positioned in the pulmonary artery. Again the pattern of appearance buildup and subsequent washout are directly related to the cardiac output. The calculations are automated.

Angiographic examination may be part of a general catheterization procedure or may be performed by itself (common in procedures carried out in a radiology department). An angiogram is a temporary "visualization" of a cardiac chamber or blood vessel by the rapid injection of a "dye" (contrast medium), which renders the chamber or blood vessel opaque to the passage of x rays as it mixes with the blood. The alteration in the x-ray pattern (temporarily increased blood x-ray density) is monitored fluoroscopically or permanently recorded by individual x-ray films recorded at fairly rapid rates (2 to 6/sec.) or on cine (movie) film at 30 to 60 frames/sec. The individual cut film or cine films, after development, can then be displayed and analyzed. The contrast medium is more or less rapidly diluted and "washed out" by the circulation and eventually excreted by the kidneys. The media are not innocuous and can cause temporary cardiac function depression, arrhythmia, pain, allergic reactions, and decrease in renal function.

There is, of course, intense interest in coronary angiography which, after a long development period, is now generally performed by inserting the catheter tip successively into the origin of both coronary arteries with manual injection of dye (5 to 8 ml) and recording the dye passage on cine film (cine coronary angiography).

When electrophysiologic studies are the catheterization objective, one or more bipolar or multipolar electrode catheters are inserted in multiple (usually) venous sites, such as both femoral veins percutaneously and a brachial vein by cutdown. Electrode catheters can be positioned in the right ventricle for pacing, across the tricuspid valve for recording the His bundle deflections, in the coronary sinus for (indirect) left atrial electrograms, and at multiple right atrial sites for electrogram recordings. Sophisticated analysis of spontaneous arrhythmia is possible using this technique. Pacing the heart is used to induce and terminate ventricular tachycardia, test anti-arrhythmic drugs, and to test the efficacy of the automatic intracardiac defibrillator (AICD, a device inserted to treat patients with life-threatening ventricular tachycardia or fibrillation or both).

Some catheterization procedures can be extensive and involve right-heart as well as the left-heart circulation, including pressure measurements, blood sampling, cardiac output determination (possibly at rest and during exercise), and multiple angiographic determinations. Such a procedure could last 2 to 3 hours. On the other hand some procedures may be quite limited, such as angiographic visualization of the abdominal aorta and lower extremity arterial circulation, which can be accomplished in 20 to 30 min.

When all the appropriate determinations have been completed, the catheter or catheters are gently withdrawn. Hemostasis is obtained (e.g., by suture of an artery, compression or ligation of a vein, or compression of the puncture site of a percutaneously inserted catheter). Finally, a small bandage is placed over the sutured cutdown site or a firm elastic bandage is placed around a percutaneous entry site. All materials coming into contact with the patient are considered to be contaminated. The patient is then carefully assisted off the catheterization table to a gurney and generally observed in an anteroom for a period of time. The procedure record is then completed, and generally a note is entered in the patient's chart describing briefly what was done and determined (if possible) and whether the patient developed particular problems or complications that need followup management.

COMPLICATIONS OF CATHETERIZATION

It is imperative for the staff to realize that elective diagnostic cardiovascular catheterization carries a small but definite mortality and morbidity risk. The procedure has clearly been made safer over the years with an overall mortality rate of 3 to 4 per 1000 cases now considered acceptable. The risk is higher when emergency procedures are undertaken and also for interventional procedures such as angioplasty.

Following are descriptions of the most important complications. Some of them are also mentioned elsewhere in the appropriate sections.

Arrhythmia. Manipulation of catheters and contrast-medium injections in the heart chambers can elicit isolated or sustained atrial or ventricular arrhythmia, which is, of course, why ECG monitoring is mandatory for cardiac catheterization. Arrhythmia occurs less frequently during peripheral angiography, as commonly performed in the radiology department. However, because a small risk remains even in these procedures, and because some patients have intrinsic arrhythmia, ECG monitoring may also be appropriate when high-risk patients undergo angiography in radiology.

Arrhythmia can occur during injection of contrast medium into the coronary arteries (coronary angiography). Bradycardia is more common but ventricle tachycardia or fibrillation or both may also occur, often following a profound bradycardia. See the section on coronary angiography in chapter 11 and the section on atropine in chapter 12.

The staff will alert the physician if rhythm disturbances develop. Sustained ventricular fibrillation requires immediate treatment. Many fatalities are a result of these types of arrhythmia.

Angina and Myocardial Infarction. Angina occurs in about 10% of patients undergoing coronary angiography. This is usually treated with nitrates in various forms (see "Nitrates" in chapter 12). If chest pain is prolonged and persistent, the patient will be admitted to the CCU and require treatment and observation for myocardial infarction (MI). The true incidence of MI, which almost always occurs in conjunction with coronary angiography, is unknown but should not exceed 2 to 3%. Cardiogenic shock may ensue if the patient sustains a major MI on the catheterization table.

Thromboembolism and Bleeding. In right-heart procedures, catheter-induced clotting and migration of thrombus, i.e., embolism (to the lung), is either rare or clinically undetected. Systemic heparinization is therefore rarely used in these procedures.

However, in left-heart or arterial procedures, blood clots (thrombus) can form around catheters and guidewires and then break off and travel (embolize) to vital organs (e.g., the brain) and cause a stroke. Rarely, thrombus in the left atrium or ventricle can dislodge and embolize.

Improvements in the surface properties of intravascular devices, such as coating guidewires with Teflon, have made these occurrences less likely to induce thrombus formation. Despite this, cardiologists routinely administer heparin systemically to further reduce this risk in left-heart procedures (see "Anticoagulants and Protamine" in chapter 12).

At the end of a procedure a residual thrombus (1 to 2%) may be at the entry side of the brachial or (less commonly) femoral artery, which can interfere with the circulation in the forearm or leg. The operator may need the assistance of a vascular surgeon in such instances.

Bleeding rarely occurs after repair of a brachial artery cutdown—total thrombosis is more likely—but considerable bleeding and hematoma formation can occur at a percutaneous femoral artery puncture site (4 to 5%). This can usually be managed by reapplication of manual pressure for a longer period (20 to 30 min.); on rare occasions surgical intervention is required.

Internal Injuries. In a small percentage of procedures, catheter tips, guidewires, needles (transseptal technique), biopsy devices, or other equipment may perforate vessel walls or heart chambers. Depending on the site, such an occurrence could produce serious or life-threatening conditions.

Perforation of a heart chamber, which results in blood leakage into the pericardium, can cause acute cardiac tamponade with shock. Immediate needle aspiration (pericardiocentesis) or surgical drainage may be necessary.

Another example of internal injury is false passage of a guidewire into the wall of the aorta (usually at the site of atheromatous plaque) with separation of the vascular wall (dissection), which is often associated with pain or, rarely, branch occlusion. Conservative management is usually adequate, but the catheterization procedure might need to be abandoned.

Other Complications. Renal failure and allergic reactions can be caused by contrast medium (see "Angiography" in chapter 11). Local or systemic infection is rare. Other rare problems are catheter knotting and the breaking off of catheter or guidewire tips. Retrieval of such fragments can be attempted with a catheter snare, but if this proves unsuccessful, surgical removal is required.

The following chapters will provide further details on all of the above briefly described aspects of catheterization.

SUMMARY

In this chapter we described, in broad outline, how a catheterization procedure is performed. Intravascular pressure and flow determinations and angiography are the most important kinds of information that we obtain. Catheters and needles are inserted by cutdown or percutaneously using local anesthesia. The x-ray machinery, incorporated in the table, allows the operator to locate the catheter tip in various circulation sites. After catheter (or needle) removal, hemostasis is obtained by direct vascular suture or pressure. The cath lab staff should also be familiar with procedure complications and be ready to assist the physician with their management.

6

Catheters and Guidewires

Cardiac catheters, and more recently guidewires, are the key instruments that are used in virtually all catheterization procedures (Fig. 6–1). They exist in a wide variety; personnel must be completely familiar with at least all those used in their laboratory. Much helpful information can be obtained by studying the sales catalogues of the major suppliers.

Catheters vary in material, which determines stiffness, configuration "memory," and tip configuration. They may also have an open or closed tip; some are designed for special purposes, such as thermal dilution cardiac output. The external end has a fitting for a syringe or stopcock and the inserted end or tip has some type of taper or special configuration.

The earliest material used for catheter construction (and still commonly used today) was woven Dacron. Such catheters are moderately flexible and, provided that they do not remain in the circulation for a long time, retain some of their original shape (memory). Extruded Dacron, used in the past, produced a rather stiff catheter, whereas extruded Teflon, though it produces a smooth slippery surface, also results in a similarly stiff catheter. A major advance was the development (by the Cordis Company) of a polyurethane (Ducor) catheter, which also has an internal braid of steel mesh wires. This resulted in a catheter with

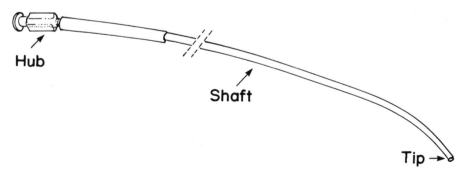

Hub

Shaft

Tip →

Fig. 6–1. Basic catheter design. The hockey-stick-like bend near the tip fascilitates movement and positioning in the various chambers and vessels.

31

excellent torque control and tip memory, and surfaces that were not excessively thrombogenic. Catheters made from polyethylene, although they have good torque control and memory, are also somewhat stiff. They have been commonly used by radiologists. The manufacturers continue to try to improve and develop new materials. A current area of development is thinner-walled catheters (of adequate strength) that can be made of a smaller caliber (so-called high-flow catheters). All catheters are impregnated with radiopaque salts of barium or analogues so that they can be visualized during fluoroscopy.

Most catheters range in size from 5 French (outer diameter 1.67 mm) to 8 French, and on occasion, 9 French.* In general, smaller-diameter catheters are used in pediatric cases but newer technologies are making available smaller catheters for larger patients as well. Catheters are approximately 100 cm in length. Much shorter ones can be used for pediatrics and some peripheral vascular angiography. 125-cm catheters are sometimes convenient for venous catheterizations from the arm.

Standard right-heart catheterization via the arm vein or percutaneously via the femoral vein is commonly performed utilizing a catheter that is provided with a single end opening cut straight or at an angle. This simple catheter, usually woven Dacron, is known as a Cournand catheter or, when thin-walled, as a Lehman catheter. A Goodale-Lubin catheter is similar but has two additional side holes near the tip (known as a "birds-eye" tip). Such catheters, after passage to the pulmonary artery, can be advanced distally to mechanically "wedge" in a small branch,

---

*French size = 3 × outer diameter (in millimeters).

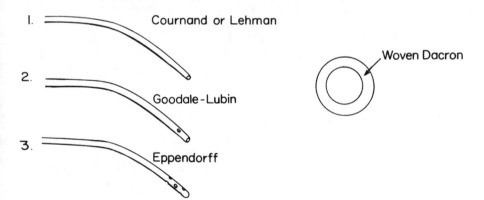

Fig. 6–2. Three types of catheters, usually constructed from woven Dacron. Types 1 and 2 are commonly used for right-heart catheterization. Type 3 is a closed-end angiographic catheter used for pulmonary angiograms, aortograms, ventriculograms, and arteriograms. Contrast medium egress is from the side holes, which reduces catheter recoil.

thereby allowing the determination of the so-called "wedge" or pulmonary capillary pressure (the analogue to the left atrial pressure) (Fig. 6–2).

Catheters designed particularly for angiography have closed ends and multiple side holes at the tip. This configuration reduces the tendency of the catheter to recoil as the bolus of contrast medium flows out at high velocity. Eppendorf and NIH catheters are constructed in this manner. Such catheters can be inserted by direct cutdown into a vein or artery or into the circulation via a sheath.

The other popular form of angiographic catheter that allows a large bolus to be injected is the so-called "pigtail" catheter (Fig. 6–3). The terminal end of the catheter is tightly looped, which inhibits the egress of dye from the end hole and promotes dye-flow from the multiple side holes. These angiographic-type catheters are used most commonly for bolus injections in the left ventricle, and also in the aorta and the right-heart chambers. A guidewire threaded through the catheter before insertion straightens the loop.

Special catheters have been developed for selective coronary angiography. The development of the modern techniques was a result of major research efforts by Sones and Judkins. The Sones catheter is constructed from woven Dacron 7 to 8 French in diameter, 80 cm long and with a long tapered tip. The catheter is inserted into the brachial artery by cutdown and, after passage to the root of the aorta, is looped in the aortic root and directed toward the orifice of one or the other coronary arteries (Fig. 6–4).

On the other hand, the Judkins approach utilizes a "pre-shaped" catheter manufactured from polyurethane or (less commonly) polyethylene, 7 or 8 French in diameter (Fig. 6–5). Newer systems are now available in smaller diameters (5 or 6 French). These catheters are inserted into the femoral artery over a

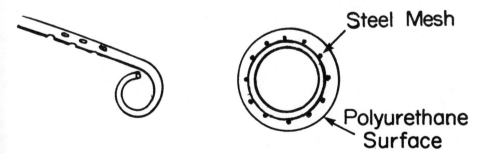

Steel Mesh

Polyurethane Surface

Fig. 6–3. *Pigtail angiographic catheter. After insertion over a guidewire, the catheter reassumes its pigtail shape. Most of the injected contrast medium finds egress from the side holes. Polyurethane provides the catheter with shape "memory"; the wire mesh supplies torque control. These are standard features of "preshaped" catheters.*

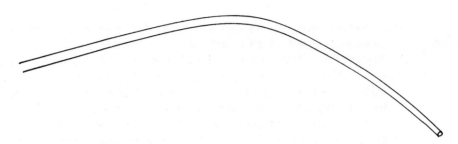

Fig. 6—4. *Sones coronary angiography catheter. Note the long tapered tip, which allows the operator to form a large loop in the aortic root.*

guidewire or via a sheath. The left coronary catheter is shaped to enter the left coronary artery; another catheter, with a different shape, is required for the right coronary artery. In most patients the 4-cm loop is utilized, but when the aortic arch is larger, a 5- or 6-cm loop is available. The Judkins catheters have a series of angles that direct the catheter into the appropriate coronary orifice. Other less commonly used preshaped catheters have been devised by Amplatz and Castillo.

In radiology there are preshaped catheters designed to enter the cerebral circulation (the so-called "head-hunter" catheters) as well as preshaped catheters for entering the celiac artery, the renal arteries, the internal mammary arteries, saphenous vein-aorto coronary bypass grafts, etc.

Judkins left

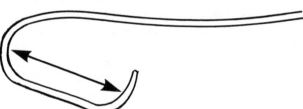

Judkins right

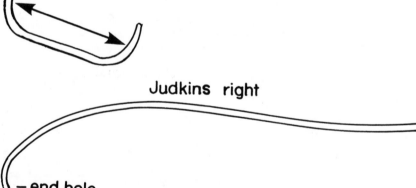

– end hole

Fig. 6—5. *The left and right coronary angiography catheters used in the percutaneous retrograde femoral technique developed by Judkins. Loops 3.5-, 4-, 5-, and 6-cm refer to the length of the primary loop of the left coronary catheter (arrow), which is selected according to the degree of dilation of the aortic root. A 4-cm loop is standard. These shapes are known as "coronary seeking.".*

Electrode catheters used for cardiac pacing or recording intracardiac electrograms (electrophysiology studies) are generally made of woven Dacron, 5 to 7 French, and usually have no lumen (Fig. 6–6). The electrodes consist of platinum rings, 2 mm wide; usually two or more are set 5 to 10 mm apart, positioned near the tip. The wire connections are contained in the wall of the catheter shaft and terminate in a pin connector. A modified electrode catheter (Myler) has a lumen and electrode rings recessed 10 cm from the tip (Fig. 6–7). With the electrodes in the right ventricle this catheter can be used in coronary angioplasty or other types of left-heart catheter procedures to protect against excessive bradycardia. This catheter also allows the monitoring of pulmonary artery pressure. Electrode catheters are inserted mainly into the right-heart chambers by brachial vein cutdown or percutaneously into the femoral vein. The electrodes are positioned in the right atrium, across the tricupsid valve, the right ventricular apex, etc.

Finally, the Swan-Ganz catheter should be mentioned.* This catheter was originally designed for cardiac monitoring in an intensive care unit setting but can also be used to advantage in the cath lab. The standard model, made of flexible polyvinyl, 120 cm long, caliber 7.5 French, has 3 lumens (Fig. 6–8). One opening is at the catheter tip; a second is 30 cm proximal to the tip. The third lumen allows manual inflation of a small balloon at the distal end of the catheter with up to 2.5 ml of air or fluid. Finally, a small thermistor (temperature-sensitive resistor) is near the tip with wire connections through the catheter wall, terminating in an electrical connection at the proximal end of the catheter.

---

*The catheter was developed by Drs. Jeremy H. Swan and William Ganz. Dr. Swan has said that he obtained the idea for the balloon flotation catheter while watching the wind fill the spinnakers of sailboats.

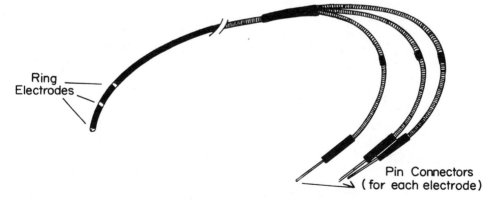

Ring Electrodes

Pin Connectors (for each electrode)

Fig. 6–6. *Example of a tripolar electrode catheter, commonly used for recording intracardiac electrograms.*

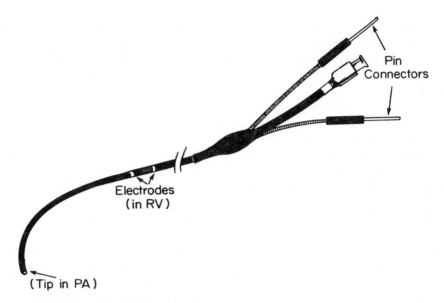

Pin Connectors

Electrodes (in RV)

(Tip in PA)

Fig. 6–7. Myler electrode catheter. The electrodes are used to pace the right ventricle; pulmonary-artery pressure can be monitored from the tip. This catheter is often used during percutaneous transluminal coronary angioplasty (PTCA).

Inflation of the balloon encourages forward passage of the catheter through the cardiac chambers by blood flow and cardiac action. Passage can be accomplished without the aid of fluoroscopy with the "blind technique" using pressure monitoring as in an ICU setting. Fluoroscopy is generally used in the cath lab to facilitate passage into the pulmonary artery, particularly when the heart is dilated. Also, inflation of the balloon with the catheter tip in the pulmonary artery functionally "wedges" the catheter tip, permitting the recording of the wedge or pulmonary capillary pressure (the analogue of the left atrial pressure). The thermistor is utilized in the thermal dilution cardiac output determination. There are a number of modifications of the basic catheter design. The Swan-Ganz catheter has been an innovative and important addition to the catheter armamentarium.

Although all labs previously reused undamaged catheters after cleaning and sterilization, commercially available catheters, except pacemaker catheters, are now specified for one-time use only.

GUIDEWIRES

Guidewires, which resemble banjo strings, are commonly available in diameters ranging from 0.018 to 0.038 in. (Fig. 6–9). Usual lengths are from 125 to 150 cm. Guidewires of 0.063 in.

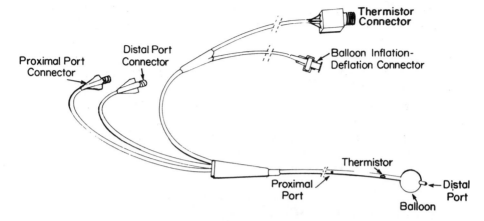

Fig. 6–8. *The Swan-Ganz catheter. It can be inserted into a vein percutaneously with the aid of a sheath or by cutdown of antecubital vein. In the cath lab it is used to determine pressure in right-heart chambers, as well as cardiac output.*

diameter are used for inserting angioplasty guiding catheters; very delicate guidewires (0.014 in.) are used in coronary angioplasty. These wires have a a steel internal core over which is

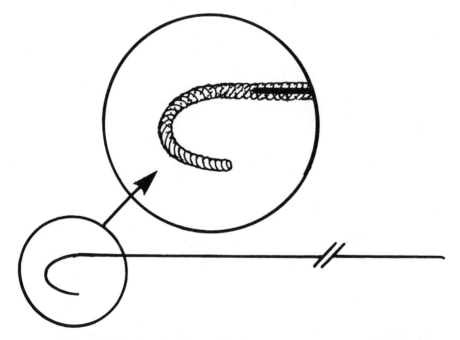

Fig. 6–9. *Standard spring guidewire, shown here with a "J" tip. The wire end that is inserted into a vessel is flexible because the stiffening core does not extend to the tip. (The "J" in this example is temporarily straightened for insertion through a cannula or catheter.)*

wound a fine steel coil or ribbon. The core generally does not extend to the distal end of the wire, resulting in a moderately "floppy" tip so that the wire easily flexes when pressed against an obstruction. A modification of the standard guidewire provides a moveable core that allows the floppy end to be lengthened or shortened at will. The tip configuration of the guidewire can be straight or a J curve of 3 to 6 mm (or larger) diameter (so-called J guidewires). Most guidewires used today are Teflon-coated, which facilitate their movement in the catheter. The surface also has a bonded heparin coating to reduce thrombogenicity. Some companies provide kits for sheath insertion that have relatively short (20 cm) uncoated steel guidewires. A guidewire with a very long floppy end has been developed to facilitate passage through tortuous vessels (Wholey wire).

Guidewires are utilized for percutaneous catheter insertion into a vein or artery, or can be preloaded into a catheter when the latter is being inserted into a sheath. Guidewires are also useful in manipulating the catheter in the vascular tree. For example, it may not be possible for the pigtail catheter to cross the aortic valve from the aorta to the left ventricle without first straightening the pigtail tip with a guidewire. Guidewires are not reused.

7

Catheter Insertion Techniques

This chapter will describe the main methods we use to insert catheters. The site chosen for insertion and the technique, cutdown or percutaneous, are determined by the objectives of the procedure, characteristics of the patient (such as age and presence of vascular disease), and the preference of the operator, which depends, to a degree, on his or her training and experience.

INSERTION BY CUTDOWN

Surgical exposure of a vein or artery is the oldest vascular access method used in catheterization. A surgical spot-light is needed. Many labs use a standing lamp equipped with a sterile lucite focusing rod that the operator can position and also turn on and off by rotating the rod up or down.

The skin incision is made in the antecubital region in adults to expose the brachial vein or artery. The arm is extended on a support attached to the edge of the catheterization table. In children or infants the saphenous vein or femoral artery/vein is exposed in the inguinal region. On rare occasions the operator may select a vessel higher up on the arm toward the axillary region and (rarely) the external jugular vein or veins in the supraclavicular area can be exposed. The skin is cleansed thoroughly with an antiseptic solution (e.g., povidone-iodine). Isolation of the site is provided by sterile towelling and sheeting or with a large sheet with a central opening.

Local anesthesia is obtained with an agent such as 1% lidocaine. The skin over the cutdown site can be anesthetized with minimal discomfort utilizing a No. 22 or 25 needle; proceeding slowly, the deeper subcutaneous tissue is then infiltrated using a slightly larger needle. To help identify a vein in the medial aspect of the antecubital fossa, generally just above the medial epicondylus, a tourniquet can be placed on the upper arm to distend the vein. If a tourniquet is used it is advisable to release it just before the anesthetic injection to avoid inadvertant puncture of the vein. Good local anesthesia will decrease the discomfort and help relax the patient. The skin incision is made with a No. 15 scalpel blade and is transverse to the course of the vessel. The midpoint of the incision, 1.5 to 3 cm in length, is centered over the vessel. Most operators utilize medium-sized curved hemostats to bluntly isolate the vein or artery. In some circumstances an assistant will be required to provide traction, or a self-retaining retractor can be used, particularly for exposure of the vessels in the inguinal region (the saphenous vein, femoral vein, and artery).

Exposure of the brachial artery (or of the femoral artery in an infant or child) is somewhat more difficult than isolating a vein. The operator makes every attempt to avoid both injury to the artery and tearing or cutting small side branches. At the same time, adequate lengths of vessel exposure are necessary to provide proper vessel control after it is opened and at the time of closure. To control bleeding, the proximal and distal ends of a vein or artery are looped with a 3-0 silk suture or umbilical tape (the latter particularly for arteries).

The venotomy or arteriotomy can be made utilizing either a fine scissors or a pointed scalpel blade (No. 11). Bleeding is controlled by traction of the proximal and distal tapes. The opening is spread with an iris forceps (or special Hahn vein dilator) and the moistened tip of the catheter is inserted.

Heparin is commonly administered for arterial catheterization to prevent clotting in or around the catheter. A standard dose would be 5000 IU injected into the distal arterial segment or into the catheter after the tip has been guided into the aorta. Heparin can also be given intravenously. The heparin is dispensed from vials containing 1000 IU/ml. The more concentrated form of heparin should not be stocked in the laboratory to avoid dosing mistakes.

Before the direct insertion of a catheter it is mandatory to purge the air from it by filling the catheter with flush solution. The proximal end of the catheter may be attached to the stopcock mechanism for continuous flushing or can be attached to a stopcock and syringe.

It is also possible to insert catheters into exposed veins or arteries that have "pigtail" tip configurations or otherwise markedly angled tips and ends. In this case a straight guidewire is inserted into the catheter, which straightens the tip configuration. It is then possible to advance the guidewire tip into the vessel followed by the catheter tip and shaft. Once the guidewire-catheter combination is advanced far enough proximally, the guidewire is withdrawn and the catheter aspirated to purge the air. Finally, it is possible to insert a vascular sheath directly into

into an exposed vein or artery. However, it is more common to insert sheaths by the percutaneous techniques (see next section).

During venous catheterization, hemostasis around the entry site is relatively easily obtained by gentle traction on the tapes. The same method may suffice for an artery, but such measures as multiple tapes in sling fashion, rubber bands, or a hemostat that supports the artery from underneath may be required. The assistants should be ready to alert the operator should excessive bleeding around the artery occur.

Removal of a straight tip catheter can be accomplished by simple withdrawal. Removal of a catheter with a contoured tip (pigtail) can be more safely achieved by reinserting a guidewire to straighten it and then withdrawing catheter and guidewire together.

Veins are managed in one of three ways after catheter removal: (1) they can be ligated, (2) they can be formally sutured when the vein is large and important (such as the femoral vein), or (3) the skin can be closed over the vein, the tapes clipped and drawn through the skin incision, and hemostatis obtained by firm pressure dressings.

Arteries are much more critical, the objective being to restore normal flow without bleeding or subsequent thrombosis. Flow is initially tested in the proximal artery by briefly relaxing the tape and allowing blood to flush. Then retrograde flow in the distal end is checked. If flow is inadequate some operators insert a 3-French Fogarty vascular balloon catheter to extract clots from the proximal or distal arterial segments. There are a variety of surgical suture techniques for the arteriotomy using 5-0 to 6-0 synthetic suture material, depending upon the preference of the operator. After surgical closure of an artery, heparin is not generally reversed with protamine. A palpable radial pulse at the wrist should be present at the termination of the arterial closure. After skin closure, a light pressure dressing is applied. The arm should be held straight for 2 to 3 hours.

PERCUTANEOUS INSERTION

Percutaneous access to the circulation, referred to as the Seldinger or percutaneous retrograde transfemoral technique, developed later than the cutdown techniques. In many laboratories the percutaneous technique has more or less supplanted the cutdown and is almost always used by radiologists. The femoral artery and vein are the vessels most commonly entered percutaneously. More recently, the technique has been used for the subclavian vein and internal jugular vein. Percutaneous entry of the brachial artery and vein is less common. The following description will mainly apply to the femoral artery, but the principle for other vessels is the same (Fig. 7–1).

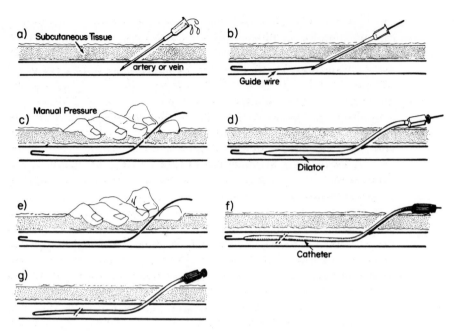

Fig. 7–1. Retrograde percutaneous catheter insertion. A. Free blood flow after vessel puncture. B. Guidewire inserted. C. Needle withdrawn, manual pressure applied to puncture side to limit blood seepage around vessel puncture site and to avoid inadvertent removal of wire. D. Insertion of vessel dilator. E. Removal of dilator, application of external pressure. F. Insertion of (end-hold) catheter over guidewire. G. Withdrawal of guidewire.

Before the procedure begins, the leg and foot are examined for signs of arterial insufficiency. An arterial bruit at the iliac or groin region, markedly reduced femoral pulsations, and reduced or absent foot pulsations might preclude the percutaneous approach. Both the dorsal pedal pulse and the posterior tibial pulse should be carefully palpated and marked with a ballpoint pen or felt tip marker for postcatheterization assessment. After skin cleansing and draping of the area the femoral artery is located by palpation, 1 to 2 cm below the inguinal ligament. Local anesthetic is introduced into the skin and subcutaneous and deep tissue overlying the vessel.

Some operators then make a small "stab wound" where the needle is to be inserted and dilate a tract in the subcutaneous tissue with a hemostat. (Alternatively, this can be done later after the guidewire has been inserted.) The puncture instrument is a No. 18 (or smaller) gauge, 2.5 in. long arterial (short bevel) cannula with removable wire needle/stylet. The needle/cannula is inserted through the stab wound (or skin) and aimed in the direction of the common femoral artery (i.e., above the profunda branch). The needle usually advances completely through the artery.

The stylet is removed from the cannula, which is then slowly withdrawn until bright red blood spurts freely. (In the case of the femoral vein the operator usually will attach a syringe to apply gentle suction and withdraw the cannula slowly until dark blood aspirates freely.) When free flow is present the flexible end of the guidewire, either straight or curved (the latter temporarily straightened with a short length of plastic tubing to fascilitate insertion), is inserted into the cannula hub and advanced centrally at least as far as the lower abdominal aorta. This is done gently, of course, to avoid damage to the vessels, and is monitored fluoroscopically to ensure that the guidewire tip is advancing properly within the vessel.

The needle is then withdrawn, leaving the guidewire in place. It is helpful to have an assistant maintain moderate pressure on the puncture site to make sure that the guidewire is not inadvertantly withdrawn and to minimize bleeding. A vessel dilator (a short length of firm, tapered Teflon tubing) is advanced over the external end of the wire, carefully tracking it through the skin and into the artery, using the wire as a guide. The dilator is then withdrawn and removed from the wire as pressure is again applied to the puncture site. Next, the catheter is threaded over the external end of the guidewire and advanced over it until the tip is at the puncture site in the skin. The guidewire is long enough, 145 to 150 cm, that its external end extends beyond the catheter's external end. The catheter tip is tapered and fits the guidewire snugly. (A variety of catheters are designed to be used this way, such as the pigtail, coronary, or multi-purpose catheters.) The catheter, with the guidewire used for tracking, is carefully advanced through the skin and subcutaneous tissue and into the artery and, under fluoroscopic control, further advanced so that the tip reaches the abdominal aorta. The guidewire is then withdrawn and the catheter is purged of air by aspiration, flushed with saline or glucose solution, and attached to a syringe stopcock assembly or the stopcock strain gauge assembly. Heparin, approximately 5000 IU, is then customarily injected intravenously or via the catheter into the abdominal aorta. After positioning the tip in the appropriate location (e.g., aortic root or left ventricle), pressure determinations and angiographic injections can then be performed.

It is possible and common to interchange catheters for different purposes. To accomplish this, a guidewire roughly 300 cm long is inserted into the catheter; the catheter is withdrawn over this guidewire, leaving a length of guidewire in the blood vessel. Again, it is necessary to maintain pressure over the puncture site during this maneuver. The next catheter is then advanced over the exchange guidewire into the vessel. The exchange guidewire can then be withdrawn and the procedure continued.

Partly because this exchange guidewire technique is cumbersome and tends to traumatize the vessel and cause bleeding, a sheath technique has been developed (Figs. 7–2 and 7–3). The sheath, which can be inserted into the artery or into the femoral, subclavian, or internal jugular veins, is essentially a semi-rigid, straw-like tube (Teflon), the outer end of which is fitted with a hemostasis valve. This prevents leakage when the sheath is in the vessel by itself (i.e., without a catheter). Most sheaths have a side arm for flushing (which can also be used for pressure recordings) attached near the external end.

After the sheath has been purged of air with flush solution, a dilator, slightly longer than the sheath, is inserted into the sheath. Then the sheath/dilator assembly is tracked over the external end of a guidewire, previously positioned in an artery or vein, and is advanced along the guidewire, through the skin and subcutaneous tissue, and into the blood vessel. First the guidewire and then the dilator is withdrawn, retaining the sheath in the artery or vein. The side arm of the sheath is aspirated and flushed and can be attached to a pressurized flush. It is then possible to insert a variety of catheters via the hemostasis valve into the vessel and exchange them at will and with ease. Most cardiac catheterization laboratories now make use of the sheath technique, although it is less commonly used in radiology departments, probably because the need to exchange catheters is less frequent. Sheaths are available from 5 French to 9 French (and larger for special purposes).

When terminating the procedure, if a sheath has not been used, the catheter is withdrawn gently. Some operators will

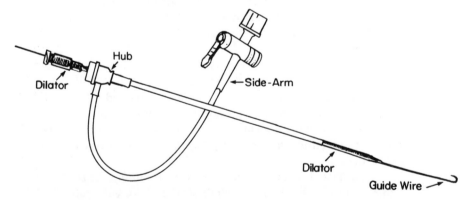

Fig. 7–2. *Standard vascular sheath that can be inserted into arteries or veins. It is available in French sizes 5 to 9 (and larger for special purposes). The hub of the sheath contains a hemostasis valve. This prevents back-bleeding, both when a catheter is inserted into the sheath and when the sheath alone is in the vessel. The caliber of the catheter used with the sheath can be the same or one French size smaller than the sheath size. (An 8-French sheath is appropriate for an 8- or 7-French catheter.)*

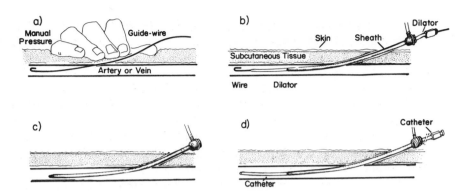

Fig. 7–3. *Insertion of vascular sheath into artery or vein. A. Guidewire in artery or vein (see Fig. 7–1 A through C). B. Sheath and dilator inserted over guidewire into vessel. C. Dilator and guidewire withdrawn. D. After aspirating blood and injecting flush solution via the sidearm of the sheath (not shown), a catheter of any tip configuration can be inserted. A pigtail catheter requires a guidewire to straighten the tip. The caliber of the catheter can be the same or one French size smaller than that of the sheath. (An 8-French sheath can be used for an 8-or 7-French catheter.)*

insert a guidewire to straighten out a pigtail catheter as it is withdrawn from the artery to reduce trauma. When a sheath has been utilized the catheter is first withdrawn from the sheath, followed by withdrawal of the sheath from the vessel. As a catheter tip or sheath is withdrawn, using two folded 4 × 4 gauze sponges, moderately firm pressure is applied over the insertion site to prevent bleeding. This pressure is generally maintained for 10 minutes or longer to prevent hematoma formation. Most operators will reverse heparin at least partially with the intravenous injection of protamine sulfate either just before removal of catheter or sheaths or immediately thereafter. (Heparin is not routinely used as an anticoagulant for venous or right-heart catheterization where thromboembolism is less of a problem.)

After hemostasis has been attained it should be possible to palpate the dorsal pedal pulse or the posterior tibial pulse or both at the previously marked site. The foot should have its original color (i.e., it should not be pale and ischemic).

A very firm elastic pressure sling is then applied. This is fashioned by using wide elastic tape: beginning from above the iliac crest, the tape is stretched down over a wad of gauze sponges at the puncture site, continuing close to the groin; the tape is then brought around the leg, up the back of the hip, and looped around anteriorly and toward the midline, thus producing a sling. This is done with the leg flexed so that when the leg is then straightened, considerable pressure is applied over the puncture site. Additional pressure can be obtained with a 5-lb sandbag. A commercial device is now available for this purpose, which is both effective and eliminates the problem of removing tape from sensitive skin, which may be hairy. The device consists of a wrap-around pelvic girdle with a broad band which is strapped around the thigh over the puncture site and attached to the girdle with Velcro.

The patient should be assisted off the catheter table and onto the stretcher so that undue straining and movement and bending of the leg does not occur. Manual pressure can be applied over the puncture site during this maneuver and when assisting the patient back into bed. Following percutaneous femoral artery catheterization, the patient should rest comfortably in bed with the leg extended for a minimum of 2 or 3 hours before standing and walking are permitted. The pressure dressing can be removed after about 4 hours and the puncture site inspected and covered with a small elastic bandage.

TRANSSEPTAL TECHNIQUE

The transseptal technique is another way of catheterizing the left-heart chambers, but it is used far less frequently than the percutaneous femoral artery or brachial-artery cutdown methods. Although the technique has undergone several modifications since its original introduction, the principle remains the same. i.e., passage of a catheter from the right atrium to the left atrium takes place by needle puncture of the interatrial septum.*

After percutaneous placement of a guidewire in the femoral vein, an 8-French sheath and dilator, similar to a standard introducer sheath but much longer (59 cm) and with a large curve at the end, is inserted over the guidewire and advanced through the inferior vena cava to the right atrium. The guidewire is replaced by a long needle, also curved at the end. When the tip of the dilator, using fluoroscopy and pressure monitoring, is against the interatrial septum, the needle is advanced beyond the dilator and through the septum and into the left atrium. It is then possible for both dilator and sheath to slide over the needle and into the left atrium. After withdrawal of the needle and dilator, the sheath remains in place and is used as a conduit to advance a curved pigtail catheter into the left atrium and across the mitral valve into the left ventricle. Pressure recordings and angiograms can be obtained in both chambers. The transseptal technique is applied in the following situations: when access to the left ventricle, in retrograde fashion from the aorta, is not possible because of severe aortic stenosis; in the presence of a tilting disc

---

*The transseptal technique was originally described by Ross and Cope in the late 1950s and further developed by Brockenbrough, Braunwald, et al. Mullins developed the currently used sheath modification.

aortic prosthesis; and (rarely) when a reliable pulmonary-artery wedge pressure cannot be recorded. Recently, the transseptal technique has been used to insert a large balloon catheter for angioplasty of the mitral valve.

Before undertaking this procedure, the patient should have prior echocardiographic assessment to ensure that there is no tumor (myxoma) or large thrombus in either atrium. Coagulation parameters should also be normal. Complications of the technique are puncture of heart or vessel walls. If only the needle causes a false puncture, the consequences are generally minor. However, advancement of the dilator and sheath (for example, into the aortic root or pericardium) could be catastrophic (leading to shock or pericardial tamponade). Thromboembolism is another potential complication. The procedure requires considerable skill and training on part of the operator.

COMPARISON OF CUTDOWN AND PERCUTANEOUS METHODS OF CATHETER INSERTION

Since there are considerable differences between these two most commonly used insertion techniques, it is important to understand their comparative advantages and disadvantages.

Direct exposure of the brachial artery or vein or both in the antecubital region permits direct insertion, if necessary, of a succession of catheters. The distance to the heart is shorter by this route and, more importantly, arteries of the upper extremities are less often the site of obstructing atherosclerotic changes than are arteries of the lower extremities. Also, it is generally easier to pass a catheter inserted into an arm vein through the right-heart chambers to the pulmonary artery than it is via the femoral vein. After removal of a catheter from the brachial artery, direct suture provides a high degree of assurance of hemostasis.

However, upper extremity vessel exposure by cutdown has certain disadvantages. Skin suturing is necessary, which requires suture removal 5 to 7 days later, and there is an incisional scar. The brachial vein and artery in some patients are small in caliber, making it difficult to insert a catheter that is large enough. Arteries may be very tortuous in the neck region, particularly in the elderly, making passage difficult or impossible. The extended arm and arm support can interfere somewhat with the rotation of the x-ray C-arm, thereby limiting angiographic projections. Because he or she is positioned closer to the x-ray source, the operator receives higher radiation exposure. Finally the technique of artery exposure and repair requires greater training and skill.

The percutaneous (modified Seldinger) technique, mostly utilized for entry into the femoral vein or artery, has many advantages. There is little scarring and no suturing. The patient's arm does not have to be extended in an immobilized position on a support, allowing the arm to be raised, temporarily if necessary, above the head. Thus, there is unimpeded freedom to rotate the x-ray C-arm around the patient's thorax and less superimposition of bony x-ray shadows in the cardiac region.

The percutaneous femoral technique is generally more quickly performed than the arm cutdown technique and has become even faster (and safer) with the development of the sheath. The technique is also more quickly learned, which is one reason why radiologists use it almost exclusively. Finally, the operator can position him or herself further from the x-ray tube and thus receives less radiation exposure.

The percutaneous technique also has disadvantages. Since it is a "blind" technique there is the possibility of vessel injury during entry and bleeding after catheter withdrawal that may not be immediately apparent. The greatest single drawback with the method is that the arteries of the lower extremities (femorals, iliacs, and lower abdominal aorta) are more frequently the site of obstructing atherosclerosis. The arteries may thus become excessively tortuous or obstructed which, despite the use of flexible guidewires, precludes catheter passage. The problem of guidewire thrombus is now minimized by Teflon-coated and heparin-bonded guide-wires and systemic heparinization.

Taking these considerations into account, the catheterization laboratory should have the capability of using either technique so that the appropriate one can be selected in a given case.

SUMMARY

In this chapter we reviewed the methods of inserting catheters into the circulation. The antecubital region is the site for exposure of the brachial artery or vein by cutdown technique. The subinguinal region is used to enter the femoral artery or vein by percutaneous technique. With the latter technique, we are aided by guidewires, dilators, and sheaths. The transeptal technique was briefly described.

The final section listed the main advantages and disadvantages of the brachial (cutdown) technique and the femoral (percutaneous) technique.

8

X-Ray Imaging

The x-ray generating and imaging equipment provides the mechanism by which we can "visualize" the internal cardiovascular structures and monitor the movement and positioning of catheters. Modern installations may now cost well in excess of $1,000,000.

The fundamental principles of an x-ray imaging system, which consists of a number of linked components, is simple. The engineering and radiation safety aspects are complex. Laboratory personnel do not need to be experts in these areas but need to understand the safe and effective utilization of the equipment. Only physicians and radiology technicians (or others under their direct supervision) may operate the equipment.

The following is a description of the x-ray installation in the Mt. Sinai Hospital, Chicago, catheterization laboratory. Many other system designs exist, some of which are simpler, others more complex.

The patient lies on a somewhat narrow, contoured, padded, stretcher-like table constructed of polycarbon, a strong radiolucent material (Fig. 8–1). The x-ray generating tube, with its shielding, is positioned under the table top. When the tube is activated, x rays travel up through the patient to enter the image intensifier tube, held in a support above the patient. This high-voltage tube converts the transmitted x rays into a small, intense visual image. A television camera is used to transmit the image to one or more TV monitors, thus providing fluoroscopy (a continuous x-ray image of a body region, such as the chest). The image can also be diverted through lenses to a camera for permanent recording on movie film (35mm cine). The cine film, after photographic processing, can then be replayed through a projector for viewing. This is known as cinefluoroscopy or cine-angiography when radiopaque contrast medium (dye) is injected while film is being exposed.

An important component in the x-ray chain is the video recorder (similar to the usual home VCRs), which makes it simple to obtain a video record of the dye injections (angiograms). This

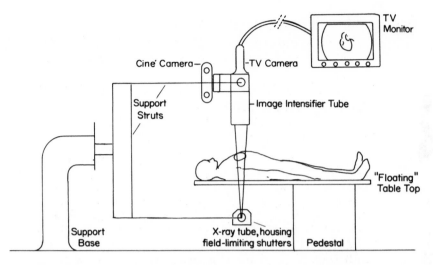

Fig. 8–1. *Diagram of basic design of cath lab x-ray installation. The table top is easily movable, even with a heavy patient, so that different parts of the heart and circulation can be shifted into the x-ray field.*

provides "instant replay," important because it may not be possible during the actual injection to assess all of the visualized structures. The cine-angiograms, available later, will provide the best detail.

One of the most important tasks of the x-ray technician is to develop exposed film, be it cine (movie-type) film or single film sheets. Most laboratories have a dedicated darkroom for this purpose. Besides feeding film into the processors and assuring proper tracking and film movement, the technician must make sure that chemicals are properly mixed and fresh, solutions are at appropriate temperature, pumps are circulating properly, etc. In addition, the technicians will label and splice film and maintain the film library.

Despite the traditional reliance on film, video and computer technology may be changing how we produce and view diagnostic quality images. New installations use high-resolution video chains (1049 lines per in. compared to the standard 525 lines per in.), creating images that rival cine-film quality. Digital storage techniques, which eliminate videotape, provide greatly improved video replay and also make possible the display of multiple angiographic frames (e.g., coronary arteries) for "road-maps." The video images can also be enhanced for optimal detail. Finally, edge-detection programs are available for analysis of coronary artery narrowings. Laser-disc systems are being developed for bulk video storage. The day of the filmless laboratory may not be far off.

The controls for the x-ray equipment are usually housed in an area adjacent to the catheterization room. The two areas are separated by a lead glass window that allows technicians and other assistants who are not required in the catheterization area to observe the procedure. Communication is aided by an intercom system.

It is possible to view an anatomic area with a 6- or 9-in. diameter field by simple switching (dual field). Newer installations can provide three field sizes. Since this is a relatively small area, the table is designed to "float" and is easily moved by releasing magnetic locks, making it possible to place different parts of the patient's anatomy in the field of exposure. Using the x-ray apparatus for fluoroscopy one readily discerns the silhouette of the beating heart against the radiolucent lung fields. Bones, because of their content of radiopaque calcium, are also clearly visible. To some degree bones block or mask the cardiovascular structures of interest.

Because of their impregnation with radiopaque salts (barium), catheters can be seen during fluoroscopy. Air injected into the balloon of a Swan-Ganz catheter appears as a radiolucency; diluted contrast medium instilled into the Swan-Ganz balloon appears as a density. Platinum electrodes on pacing catheters and metallic markers at strategic points on balloon dilitation catheters are also easily discernible.

Angiographic principles (contrast medium or dye enhancement of cardiac chambers or vessels) will be discussed in chapter 11.

The x-ray tube and image-intensifying tubes, below and above the patient respectively, produce a PA (posterior-anterior) projection that has a somewhat small field size (approximately twice the projected area of the normal heart). It has already been mentioned that head, foot, and lateral movement is easily attained with the floating table top, thereby permitting the field to cover almost the entire body. Also important is the ability to rotate the x-ray tube and image tube radially around the thorax of the patient in excess of 180° (Fig. 8–2). This capability allows visualization of the heart and blood vessels in oblique and lateral projections, which greatly facilitates analysis of anatomy and function, particularly during angiography.

In addition, the apparatus allows for cranial and caudal angulation simultaneous with radial angulation, as described above, which enhances the demonstration of otherwise overlapping structures. This is most crucial for coronary angiography (Fig. 8–3).

By using two independent systems, it is possible to obtain flouroscopy or angiography simultaneously in two planes, for example, PA and lateral. In this way when contrast media is injected into the left ventricle, two views of the chamber can be obtained with one injection.

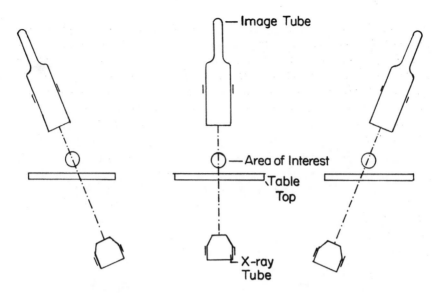

Fig. 8–2. Diagram of the capability to rotate the support system around the patient's body and thereby obtain oblique and lateral x-ray projections, which is important in many types of angiography (e.g., that of the left ventricle and coronary arteries).

Another format for permanently recording images (essentially angiograms) is the use of film changers (Fig. 8–4). In this mode (called serialography), instead of beaming the x rays through the patient and into the image intensifier, the patient and equipment are oriented so that the x rays, after passing through the patient, impinge upon and expose standard individual x-ray film sheets, which are moved serially through the changer at a rate of 1 to 6/sec. Such "cut-film" angiogram systems are commonly used in x-ray departments and produce large, easily viewed, and finely detailed images of heart chambers, the pulmonary artery, the aorta and branches, etc.

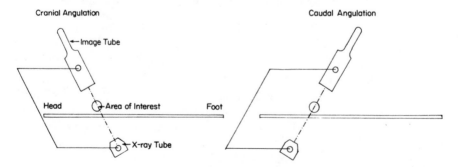

Fig. 8–3. Diagram of the capability to angle the system that supports the image tube and x-ray tube in a cranial or caudal direction. This is especially important in coronary angiography, because the coronary arteries (and obstructive lesions) can radiographically overlap in nonangulated projections.

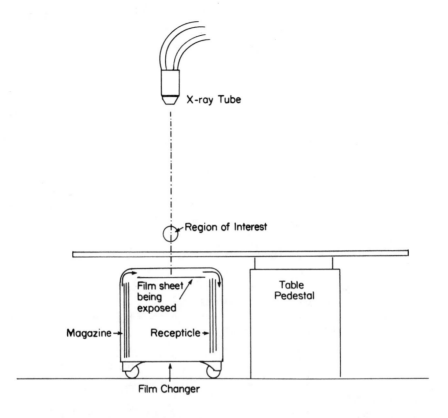

Fig. 8—4. Equipment used for "rapid-film" angiographic technique. Film sheets are transported from the magazine (on the left) to intensifier screens at the top (under the patient) and, after a synchronized x-ray exposure, transported to the receptacle (on the right). The exposure rate can vary from 1 to 6 per sec., and a total of 30 film sheets can be exposed. The system is activated when contrast medium is injected and is circulating in the region of interest (such as the lungs, heart, or aorta). After the exposures are completed, the technician removes the film receptacle and develops the film in an automatic processor.

Finally, the x-ray table can be programmed to periodically move the patient along as the contrast medium circulates through the body. For example, dye injected into the abdominal aorta circulates to the lower extremities. The initial serialographic filming may begin in the abdominal aorta. The table then moves the patient so that the pelvic region and then the knees and legs, in sequence, are in the x-ray path as the dye circulates toward the feet. Again a single injection of dye suffices for imaging multiple areas of the body.

RADIATION SAFETY

Diagnostic radiation, when properly used, poses little risk to patients. However, laboratory personnel working in a radiation environment need to understand and practice precautionary measures. The equipment in use today is far safer than that used in first-generation laboratories. This is mainly because the development of image intensifiers has permitted a drastic lowering of radiation dose (with attendant reduction of radiation to the patient as well).

X rays scatter ("secondary" radiation) from the x-ray tube, table, and patient and spread widely around the room. Tube scatter is contained by steel or lead housing. Lead shielding can, to some extent, be draped around the patient to reduce scatter radiation. The laboratory walls are lead lined. Most importantly, three main safety operating principles must be observed: expose x ray for the briefest periods of time, columnate (narrow the field) as much as possible, and stand as far as possible from the x-ray source.

However, no measures such as the above can prevent all x-ray scattering from reaching laboratory personnel. Therefore, it is mandatory that all personnel in the laboratory during x-ray exposure wear lead-lined aprons and face the x-ray source. Those working close to the source may also wear lead collars to protect the thyroid gland and leaded glasses to protect the eyes. Leaded glass shields are available for the protection of those working close to the patient, as are large lead panels behind which personnel may stand during moments of high radiation such as angiography.

Finally, all personnel are required to wear x-ray film badges, one underneath the apron and one worn near the neck region, for individual monitoring of x-ray exposure. Radiation exposure to personnel is a clear-cut hazard. Although this hazard, with appropriate precautions, can be reduced to a safe minimum, it cannot be eliminated altogether. This is mainly why usual policy excludes known pregnant personnel from working directly in the lab.

To obtain optimal function and safe operation, the x-ray equipment requires periodic preventive maintenance and radiation checks. The latter assures that there is no inappropriate radiation leakage beyond the imaging field and that the machinery is operating according to manufacturer's specifications and radiation safety agency guidelines.

SUMMARY

The way we use the x-ray equipment in the catheterization laboratory should now be understood. Operation is fairly simple; only the technology is complex. Safety precautions are required.

9

Intracardiac and Intravascular Pressure Determinations and Recordings

Physiologists in the mid-19th century studied intravascular pressure in animals. The more recent development of clinical cardiac catheterization has shown that cardiac and intravascular pressure determinations are of great importance because alterations in hemodynamics are indicators of abnormal structure and function.

From recordings taken at or near the tip of a catheter (or from a needle) it is possible to determine pressure at virtually any site in the circulation. Although miniature pressure transducers can be mounted at the catheter tip, most pressure determinations are recorded using the catheter as a fluid-filled column to transmit the pressure, via tubing and stopcocks to a strain gauge.* (Fig. 9–1). The upper part of this device consists of a fluid chamber in the shape of a hemisphere, about 1.5 ml in volume. The base of the hemisphere is sealed with a thin flexible membrane. This membrane is coupled against a flat metal plate by a few drops of fluid. Pressure changes in the upper chamber (when closed to room air pressure by a stopcock), transmitted from the catheter, cause vibratory movement of the metal plate. The plate is part of an electronic circuit that creates voltages proportional to the plate movement. Other electronic circuitry then amplifies and displays the resultant waveforms for monitoring and permanent recording. It is of the utmost importance to purge the tubing and strain-gauge chamber of air bubbles, as these bubbles degrade and dampen the waveform signals. The fluid-chamber section of the strain gauge is sterile (now usually disposable), whereas the electronic component can be reused indefinitely if not damaged.

Pressure measurements are made with reference to the level of the heart (mid axillary line) as the zero reference point.

---

*The strain gauge, also known as a pressure transducer, converts the mechanical pressure waves into electric signals.

55

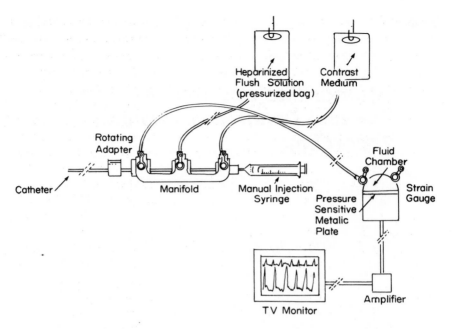

Fig. 9–1. Diagram of the simplified manifold, tubing, and strain-gauge system (preferred by the author). The stems of the manifold stopcocks point to the "closed" or "off" position. (In the diagram the manifold is set for injection of dye or flush solution into the catheter). The 24-in. semi-rigid (pressure) tubing leads from the strain-gauge, which is mounted on a side-rail of the x-ray table, to port No. 1 of the manifold. Heparinized flush solution, hanging on a bracket above the table is connected by tubing to port No. 2 of the manifold. Contrast medium in a glass container is also hung on a bracket and is tubed to port No. 3. A control syringe (10 ml) is attached to the end of the manifold. The catheter hub is attached to the rotating adapter at the other end. The electronic signal induced in the strain-gauge by pressure fluctuations in the circulation travel via cable to an amplifier and are displayed on a monitor.

Therefore, after the patient is positioned on the catheterization table, the technician or nurse raises or lowers the bracket holding the strain gauge according to the size and position of the patient. Standard practice requires periodic testing of the electronic calibration of the strain gauge against a mercury manometer reference. The display and recording of pressure and other waveforms are controlled from a console-like recorder usually located in the area adjacent to the catheterization room. The nurse or technician operating the recorder is thus protected from scatter radiation. The recorder houses a group of electronic amplifiers, which are connected by cables to the pressure transducers and other electronic signals (ECG) derived from the patient. The amplified signals are displayed on a CRT (cathode-ray tube), an oscilloscope, or (more recently) a video-type screen. Up to three or four pressure waves (each requiring a separate catheter, tubing, strain gauge, and amplifier system) may be displayed simultaneously (e.g., left ventricular, wedge, and femoral artery pressures). The electrocardiogram is always shown. "Slave" scopes are mounted in the catheterization room for viewing by physician(s) and other personnel working in that area.

Permanent records are made with a strip chart recorder. This produces a time-base graph on light sensitive paper that is chemically or heat processed for immediate viewing as the strip (approximately 6 in. wide) emerges from the device. The wave forms can then be analyzed in detail.

Before the permanent physiologic pressure wave form (e.g., left ventricular) is actually recorded, it is first necessary to record a calibration signal. This is obtained from the amplifier/strain-gauge combination and plots various pressure levels (e.g., 20, 50, and 100 mmHg) on the graph, against which the pressure waves from the patient can be measured. (This is similar to the 1 cm/1 mm volt calibration on the ordinary electrocardigraph.)

Some laboratories utilize computers for "on-line" pressure wave-form acquisition analysis and generation of tabular reports. The nurse or technician is trained to enter patient information into the computer and initiate the report process. Table 9–1 shows normal pressure values.

Table 9–1. *Normal Intracardiac and Intravascular Pressure Valves*

Site	Pressure (mmHg)
Right atrium (RA, "CVP")	2-6 (mean)
Right ventricle (RV)	25-30 systolic 2-6 end diastolic
Pulmonary artery (PA)	30-35 systolic 10-12 diastolic 15 (mean)
Left atrium (LA)	6-12 (mean)
Left ventricle (LV)	120-130 systolic 10-12 end diastolic
Aorta (Ao)	120-130 systolic 80 diastolic 92 (mean)

Detailed discussion of pressure wave forms is beyond the scope of this book. However, a working knowledge of the basic principles will greatly enhance the cath lab worker's understanding of the nature and importance of the information being acquired. The following description pertains to patients ordinarily encountered in the catheterization laboratory and not those with acute conditions such as shock and acute myocardial infarction, as encountered in the ICU.

1. The right atrial (RA) pressure is also known as the central venous pressure (CVP in ICU parlance). It represents the filling pressure of the right ventricle. Elevations of the RA pressure occurs in fluid-overload states, stenosis (in congenital heart disease), or insufficiency of the tricuspid valve. RA pressure is also elevated when diastolic right ventricular (RV) pressure (often referred to as the end diastolic pressure, or RV-EDP) is increased. The latter can occur when there is abnormal myocardial function (toxic or ischemic) or when excessive systolic pressure (systolic overload) of the RV is present.

2. Right ventricular systolic pressure increases in response to either obstruction of the RV outflow tract (pulmonic stenosis, which is generally congenital), increased resistance to flow in the pulmonary circuit (artery) (pulmonary hypertension), or when there is communication between the right and left ventricles (ventricular septal defect).

3. Pulmonary artery pressure increases when there is diffuse pulmonary vascular obstruction (diffuse pulmonary embolization) or lung tissue damage. However, elevated pulmonary artery pressure is most commonly caused by increased pulmonary capillary pressure (PCP) or "wedge" pressure due to abnormal structure or function in the left-heart chambers. The PCP is the convenient analogue of left atrial pressure. (The left atrium is the cardiac chamber least accessible to direct catheterization.) Obstruction of the outflow of the left atrium into the left ventricle, as with mitral stenosis, elevates left atrial pressure.

4. Elevation of the diastolic pressure in the left ventricle (commonly referred to as the end diastolic pressure, or LV-EDP) is the most common reason for the increase in left atrial pressure (and thereby wedge and pulmonary artery pressure), and generally signifies (left) heart dysfunction. Examples of pathologic processes that damage and reduce left ventricular myocardial function are ischemic scarring (coronary artery disease), toxic damage, (such as that from alcohol), and abnormalities of the mitral and aortic valves. The pressure in the left ventricle can be measured directly, most often with a catheter passed retrograde from the aorta.

5. The most common cause of elevated systolic pressure in the left ventricle is systemic arterial hypertension. When the aortic valve is normal, systolic blood pressure, determined with the usual cuff manometer, is the same as the left ventricular systolic pressure.

However, when the outflow of the left ventricle is obstructed, as with stenosis of the aortic valve, the systolic pressure in the left ventricle is higher than the arterial systolic pressure—by as much as 100 mmHg in severe cases. This is known as a "gradient". Eventually, systolic overload of the left ventricle results in increased diastolic pressures and hemodynamic dysfunction or failure with a cascade effect on the rest of the circulation.

SUMMARY

The determination of pressures in various sites of the circulation provides important clinical information concerning structure and function. Catheters transmit the pressure wave forms to strain gauges for electronic conversion and amplication. These wave forms are monitored and analyzed manually or by computer, and can be permanently recorded. Knowledge of normal intracardiac and vascular pressures and the typical abnormalities will enhance the understanding of the procedures and improve work performance.

10

Cardiac Output and Shunt Detection

The heart is the pump that drives blood through the circulation. We use the term cardiac output, in liters per minute, to denote the amount of circulated blood. For example, if with each beat the heart ejects 70 ml and there are 70 beats per min., the cardiac output is 4900 ml or 4.9 l/min. An intimate feedback relationship exists between the peripheral vasculature and the heart, one that determines pressures and flow rates. This chapter will describe the concepts underlying the measurement of cardiac output. It is also appropriate here to discuss intra-cardiac shunts and their detection.

CARDIAC OUTPUT

The basis of all clinical cardiac output determinations is the so-called Fick principle, which states that in a closed steady-state system, in this case the heart and blood vessels, the amount of an indicator flowing into the system equals the amount of indicator flowing out of the system. The Fick principle can be utilized in one of two ways. In the first, the classic cardiac output by "Fick," oxygen is used as the "indicator." The second method is a modification of the Fick principle, utilizing it in the form of an indicator dilution technique (IDT). In the original IDT, a color dye (e.g., indocyanine green) was injected into the circulation. Although still in use in some laboratories, the dye indicator has been replaced with a thermal indicator (cold-fluid injection). The thermister at the tip of the Swan-Ganz catheter determines the temperature fluctuations induced in the blood.

In patients with more advanced states of heart failure the cardiac output can be decreased to about one half the normal value. In hyperkinetic states, such as anemia and hyperthyroidism, the cardiac output increases.

60

It is also possible to determine the cardiac output in an exercising patient. Exercise is performed by attaching a bicycle ergometer to the foot end of the table with the patient's feet placed on the pedals. Typically, a normal individual can easily double the baseline cardiac output whereas the patient with a failing heart may show virtually no increase. (Pressure measurements during exercise are also important).

Normal values for cardiac output at rest are between 5 and 8l/min. The cardiac index, obtained by dividing cardiac output by square meters of body surface area, allows comparison between patients of different sizes. The normal cardiac index ranges from 2.75 to 3.50 l/min./m² body surface area. Cardiac output is also used in the derivation of other data such as aortic and mitral valve area, vascular resistance, and stroke volume and work, which provide additional information about cardiovascular function.

CARDIAC OUTPUT DETERMINATION BY FICK

Cardiac output by this method requires three pieces of data: the amount of oxygen taken up by the body (oxygen consumption), the oxygen content in the arterial blood (not to be confused with arterial blood gases, which are ordinarily expressed in terms of mmHg), and the oxygen content in the mixed venous blood, which is ordinarily sampled from the pulmonary artery. The difference in oxygen content between the arterial blood and the pulmonary artery blood is known as the arteriovenous (A-V) oxygen difference. Utilizing a simple algebraic formula, the A-V difference and oxygen consumption provides the value of cardiac output (CO):

$$CO = \frac{O_2 \text{ Consumption}}{10 \text{ (Arterial } O_2 \text{ Content} - \text{Mixed Venous } O_2 \text{ Content)}}$$

where CO is l/min., O_2 consumption is in ml/min. BTPS (body temperature and pressure, saturated), and arterial and venous O_2 content is in ml/100 ml blood. The expression in the denominator is the A-VO$_2$ difference.

For example, assume the following data:

O_2 Consumption = 250 ml/min.
Arterial O_2 Content = 19 ml/100 ml blood
Venous O_2 Content = 14 ml/100 ml blood

Then

$$CO = \frac{250}{10 \ (19 - 14)} = \frac{250}{50} = 5 \text{ l/min.}$$

Arterial blood can be withdrawn into a heparinized syringe from either a cannula in a peripheral artery or a catheter in the aorta or the left ventricle. When taken from a catheter for analysis, 2 or 3 ml of blood must first be withdrawn with a syringe from the "dead space" of the catheter; a fresh heparinized syringe is then attached to aspirate the blood sample. This ensures appropriate sampling from the desired site.

The usual method of oxygen consumption determination is to allow the patient to breathe through a mouthpiece and collect the expired air. The collection chamber can be a large tank (Tissot spirometer) or a Douglas gas bag. The expired air collection is obtained over several minutes' time. When using the Tissot spirometer, the patient's expired air is first used to "wash out" the residual air in the spirometer (e.g., 3 min.-washout three times), followed by a 3-min. collection of the final specimen. The "wash-outs" are not necessary when using the Douglas bag. In any case, a period of quiet, "steady-state" breath collection is required to obtain a representative sample. The laboratory technician measures the exact volume of the expired air (ml/min.), (Scholander or polarigraphic method), analyzes a sample and makes the calculations necessary to derive oxygen consumption.

There are also several ways by which the blood can be analyzed for oxygen content (O_2 saturation and hemoglobin method or Van Slyke determinations). Determined values of the cardiac output, taken in conjunction with pressure data, can be used to derive other useful information such as aortic or mitral valve area, pulmonary or systemic vascular resistance, and stroke work.

Two important considerations make the Fick method less than ideal. The first is that because expired air must be collected the patient must be conscious, cooperative, and not agitated. The second is that this method is labor-intensive, requiring considerable skill on the part of one or more technicians.

CARDIAC OUTPUT DETERMINATION BY THERMAL DILUTION TECHNIQUE

This method utilizes a transiently induced decrease in blood temperature as a "thermal" indicator. The technique became practical with the development of the Swan-Ganz balloon flotation catheter. When this catheter is properly positioned the tip lies in the main right or left pulmonary artery branch and the proximal port opens into the right atrium. A tiny bead thermistor (a rapidly responding temperature-measuring device) is mounted close to the catheter tip; the device is capable of tracking fluctuations in blood temperature almost instantaneously. Cardiac output is determined by rapidly injecting, with a syringe, a 5-or 10-ml bolus of saline or 5% dextrose into the RA via the catheter. Room-temperature or, better, iced solution is used. The circulation transports the "cold" indicator to the pulmonary artery, resulting in a transient fall of blood temperature at the thermistor site (in the PA), the extent of which depends on the cardiac output. Automatic calculations are obtained with a simple bedside computer. To make the determination, the computer requires the following information:

1. Injectate volume (usually 5 or 10 ml)
2. Thermistor calibration factor (supplied by catheter manufacturer)
3. Injectate temperature (measured with a good laboratory thermometer or, as is now possible and much more convenient, a second thermistor, attached to the injection syringe/stop-cock system; this provides the computer with the exact temperature of the injectate as it enters the catheter).

The theory of the thermal dilution cardiac output, although not difficult, is beyond the scope of this book.

At least three bolus injections (as rapidly as possible) and determinations are made. Three close values are averaged. If one value varies widely an additional one or two can be obtained. The skills required by the technicians to determine cardiac output by IDT are less demanding than those required for the standard Fick.

INTRA-CARDIAC SHUNT DETECTION

Normal blood flow after birth can be considered to take place in tubes and chambers connected in series. This unidirectional flow system can be diagrammed thusly:

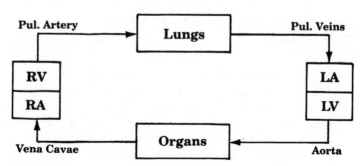

Flow is in the direction of the arrows.

In simple cases, we speak of intracardiac shunts as flow (in either direction) between the atria (atrial septal defect), the ventricle, (ventricular septal defect), or between the aorta and pulmonary artery (persistent ductus arteriosis).

Diagramatically, an atrial septal defect appears thusly:

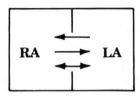

Flow may be from left atrium to right atrium (left to right shunt), from RA to LA (right to left shunt), or bidirectional. Similar flow abnormalities exist for other sites. (The pressure and angiographic abnormalities that occur in the presence of shunts will not be discussed.)

The usual cause of intracardiac shunting is congenital (congenital heart disease), with clinical manifestations occurring early in life (large ventricular septal defect) or sometimes only after 30 to 40 years (atrial septal defect). Abnormal intracardiac connections may be associated with valve obstructions, hypoplastic chambers, and abnormally connected arteries and veins to produced complex anomalies. Cyanosis (arterial blood oxygen desaturation) is common, caused by desaturated venous blood entering the arterial circulation.

Occasionally we encounter intracardiac shunting after trauma (stab wound or bullet injuries).

In the catheterization laboratory, shunt detection is usually accomplished by analyzing the blood for oxygen saturation (or content) at various sites. Another way to detect shunts is based on indicator dilution techniques whereby an indicator (e.g., indocyanin green, ascorbic acid, or hydrogen), when injected into the circulation, demonstrates a typical abnormal flow pattern. Only the O_2 saturation technique will be described.

To illustrate, we can consider a 5-year-old child with a persistent ductus arteriosus. This is a tubular structure that connects the aorta near the take-off of the subclavian arterial to the pulmonary artery. It functions in fetal life and ordinarily closes shortly after birth. We will assume left-to-right flow, that is, from aorta to pulmonary artery, because pulmonary vascular resistance is low (before the onset of permanent changes in the pulmonary vasculature from chronic excess flow).

To demonstrate and quantify the abnormal flow, a right-heart catheterization (percutaneous technique via the femoral vein or by saphenous vein or femoral vein cut down) is performed with insertion of a pediatric NIH or Eppendorf catheter. Blood is withdrawn with the catheter tip fluoroscopically located in the inferior and superior vena cavae, the right atrium, the right ventricle, and both branches of the pulmonary artery. Blood is also sampled from a peripheral artery (needle puncture). To obtain proper samples, 2 to 3 ml blood must first be withdrawn from the catheter with a syringe to "wash out" the dead space of the catheter. Then a second heparinized syringe is attached for withdrawal of 3 to 5 ml for O_2 saturation determination. The syringe must be clearly labeled to show the site of blood origin. (The blood from the "washout" syringe can be reinjected before taking the next sample.)

Results typical (though somewhat idealized) of a ductus would be shown in Table 10-1.

Table 10-1. *Typical results of a ductus.*

Site	O_2 Saturation (%)
Inferior vena cava	78
Superior vena cava	72
Right atrium	75
Right ventricle	75
Right pul. artery	88
Left pul. artery	88
Femoral artery	96

The SVC blood is slightly less saturated than the IVC blood (venous blood from the brain, draining into the SVC, is relatively desaturated; venous blood from the kidneys, draining into the IVC, is relatively highly saturated). Caval flows mix in the right atrium with coronary sinus blood to average about 75% O_2 saturation. The same saturation exists in the RV. Our example now shows a large increase in O_2 saturation in the pulmonary artery blood, i.e., an O_2 saturation "step-up" caused by the flow of fully oxygenated blood (95% saturation) from the aorta into the pulmonary artery. This mixes with blood entering the pulmonary artery from the RV and results in a final saturation of 88% (other aspects of the diagnosis of the ductus will not be discussed).

Using the data, it is possible to obtain a quantification of the amount (volume flow) of the shunt flow. In its simplified form, the formula for pulmonary/systemic blood flow ratio is as follows:

$$\frac{\text{Arterial } O_2 \text{ Saturation } - \text{ Mixed Venous Blood Saturation Proximal to Shunt}}{\text{Arterial } O_2 \text{ Saturation } - \text{ Mixed Venous Blood Saturation Distal to Shunt}}$$

Entering the data, we obtain*

$$\frac{96 - 75}{96 - 88} = \frac{21}{8} = 2.6$$

This means that blood flow in the lungs is 2.6 times greater than in the systemic circulation, which represents a shunt of moderate size. A large shunt would have a ratio of greater than 3 to 1 and a small shunt of less than 1.5 to 1. Actual flow rates (1/min.) can be calculated if cardiac output is known. The technique is sensitive to shunt ratios as low as 1.2 to 1.3 to 1. Indicator dilution techniques are even more sensitive. A direct intravascular oxymeter, mounted on a catheter, can also be used, obviating the need to withdraw blood samples.

Patients with other types of shunts are studied in an analogous manner. During the procedure, or immediately thereafter, the laboratory technician or, less frequently, the nurse, will analyze each of the samples for O_2 saturation using an oxymeter or derive O_2 saturations from blood gas analysis. Great care must be taken to avoid mislabeling the origin of the blood sample.

SUMMARY

Cardiac output determination is an important component of many catheterization procedures. Decreased cardiac function is often associated with decreased cardiac output. The main methods in use today are the Fick cardiac output, in which oxygen is the "indicator," and the thermal dilution application of the indicator dilution technique. The method used depends upon the equipment available, the skill of the technicians, the condition of the patient, and the experience of the physician.

Shunt detection and quantification are usually undertaken in patients with congenital heart disease. Oxygen saturation determinations, at various locations in the heart and great vessels, are used (along with other methods) in diagnosing this condition.

---

*In this illustration the pulmonary artery is considered distal to the shunt (i.e., receives shunt flow), and the other right-heart structures are proximal to the shunt (i.e., do not receive shunt flow).

11

Angiography

Angiography is an essential component of the cardiovascular catheterization procedure. It reached full development somewhat later than the techniques for pressure and flow determinations and yields important information of a fundamentally different kind.

The blood pool in vessels and the cardiac chambers is not "visible" during fluoroscopy. Angiography is the process whereby contrast medium (the so-called "dye"), injected into the blood, causes the blood to appear as a density, or radiopaque area, in the radiographic (x-ray) field. We are thus able to "see" the silhouette of the vessel or cardiac chamber containing the radiopaque blood (Figs. 11–1 and 11–2). An assessment can be made of such factors as the size of a chamber, whether an artery is stenosed or occluded, and, in the case of the left or right ventricle, whether the vigor of contraction is normal or diminished. The circulation rapidly dilutes the dye (i.e., "washes" it away), which means that only several seconds are available for x-ray imaging after dye installation.

In the radiology department vascular angiography, by itself, is a common procedure. In the catheterization laboratory angiography is almost always incorporated into a procedure that includes pressure and flow measurements.

CONTRAST MEDIA

The solutions owe their radiopacity to atoms of iodine coupled to an organic molecule.* Compared to blood, the solutions are 8 to 10 times more viscous, ionized, and highly hypertonic. (HOCM stands for "high osmolality contrast media." See below for discussion of the newer non-ionic contrast media). The iodine

---

*A commonly used preparation is a 76% solution of sodium-diazotrate (10%) and methylglucamine-diazotrate (66%). The iodine molecules are linked to the diazotrate (370 mg I/ml). A 50% solution can be used for cerebral and limb angiography.

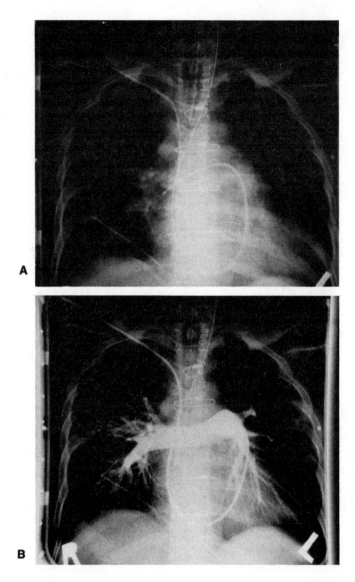

Fig. 11–1. Pulmonary angiogram. A. "Scout" x-ray film of chest (i.e., a film taken before injection of contrast medium) showing thoracic skeleton, lung fields, and heart, as well as miscellaneous postoperative wires and clips. An angiographic catheter has also been introduced via an arm vein (not shown) and tracked through the right atrium and right ventricle, with the tip positioned in the pulmonary artery (right branch). B. Contrast medium ("dye") has been injected and a film exposed about 2 sec. later. (Actually, there is a series of rapid film exposures.) The right and left pulmonary arteries and secondary branches are now "visible." The purpose of this angiogram was to attempt to identify emboli (blood clots) in the pulmonary vasculature. This diagnosis is made when pulmonary arterial branches are not "visualized" (clots are preventing flow of dye into the branches) or the vessel contours are irregular ("filling defects"). In this case, the study was considered normal. (Considerable detail is lost in reproduction.)

content is mostly responsible for allergic reactions (e.g., urticaria, bronchospasm, and, fortunately rarely, laryngospasm). Prior skin testing of the patient is not a routine practice. However, in most laboratories a small test dose (0.5 to 1 ml) of the dye is injected into the circulation at the site where the subsequent larger injection will be made. The patient is then observed for adverse reaction for several minutes.

When there is a history of a minor dye reaction (e.g., mild itching or minimal urticaria) the patient may be pretreated with antihistamines. With a history of a major dye reaction, it is probably best to avoid angiography altogether unless it is critically important to the management of a serious cardiovascular condition. In such a case the patient is commonly pretreated with corticosteroids and antihistamines.

Another undesirable effect of the dye is a variable degree of local pain, associated with vasodilation, particularly when the injection occurs in a smaller artery (e.g., the femoral or carotid artery). When a large bolus injection is made (e.g., into the aortic root) the patient develops a general sensation of warmth and may experience a headache or flushed sensation. This unpleasant state usually dissipates in about 10 sec. The patient should be forewarned to expect these temporary effects.

Dye that circulates through the heart or is injected directly into the coronary circulation causes some degree of myocardial depression. The pain and vasodilation action as well as some of the cardiac depression effect is caused by the high osmolality content of the medium. The direct cardiac effects usually manifest themselves as transient bradycardia and hypotension (caused by vasodilation and decreased cardiac output).

Finally, because the dye is excreted by the kidneys, decreased renal function may occur after an angiographic examination in patients with previously compromised renal function. This can be counteracted to some degree by adequate I.V. hydration. Thus, the angiographer has to consider a number of adverse dye effects in planning a procedure for a given patient.

The angiographic contrast media in use today are far safer than those available originally. Nevertheless, persistence of the side effects has led to efforts to produce superior formulations. This has been achieved by linking the (three) iodine atoms to newly developed organic compounds, solutions of which are non-ionized and therefore have a much lower osmolality.*

Several products of this type, commonly known as non-ionic or low osmolality angiographic contrast media (LOCM), are

---

*Standard contrast media used for cardiac and coronary angiography has an osmolarity of 1940 (m Osm/kg H_2O) compared to 796 (m Osm/kg H_2O) for the newer non-ionic preparations.

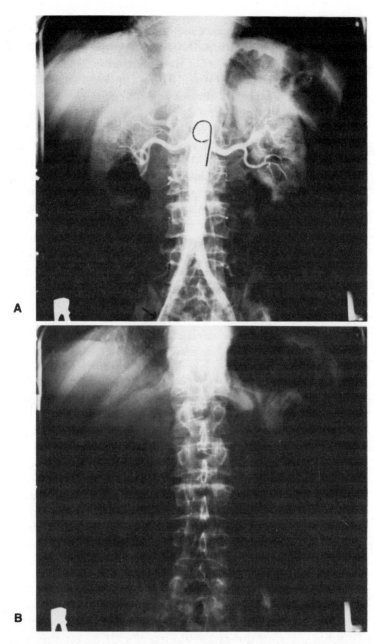

Fig. 11–2. Abdominal aortogram. A. Scout film, before injection of contrast medium, of the lower abdomen showing vertebral column and upper pelvic bones. B. A pigtail catheter has been inserted from the right femoral artery and advanced into the abdominal aorta. (The loop of the catheter is redrawn because of masking by the contrast medium; the lower shaft of the catheter is indicated by the arrow.) This exposure, made 1.6 sec. after the start of the contrast-medium injection, shows the "visualized" inner contours of the abdominal aorta, the renal arteries, and the iliac arteries. No obvious abnormalities are present.

available and are generally acknowledged to have fewer or less drastic side effects. Angiographers are in clear agreement that with the use of the new agents patients experience much less pain (especially with venography and peripheral angiography), nausea, and flushing. The major drawback of the non-ionic agents is that they now cost up to five to eight times as much as the traditional products. Increased use will undoubtedly occur when the cost decreases.

IMAGING FORMATS

There are two commonly used x-ray imaging formats: the large size, so-called "cut-film" technique and the image intensifier cine (movie) technique, whereby 35mm cine film is exposed at 30 to 60 frames/sec. (For further discussion of imaging techniques, see chapter 8.)

The cut-film format is more appropriate when movement of the anatomic structure being imaged is minimal. Therefore, this format is utilized, for example, in pulmonary angiography and aortography. Detail is excellent.

The cine technique is better adapted to imaging more rapidly moving structures such as the left ventricle and the coronary circulation.

POWER INJECTORS

Depending on the purpose of the angiograms, rapid injections of a large volume of contrast media may be required (e.g., 50 ml delivered in 3 sec.—the so-called bolus injection). Because of the high viscosity of the contrast media and the flow resistance in the catheter, manual injection is impossible; therefore, a power or pressure injector is required. Modern injectors are electrically driven and have sophisticated controls for injecting specific volumes at specific flow rates. Pressure generation can reach 500 to 600 lbs/inch^2.

The injector is filled by sterile aspiration from the dispenser container, using sterile plastic tubing. Air is purged from the syringe and tubing before making the connection to the catheter. After all connections are checked and found to be tight, some blood can be aspirated back into the syringe to ensure that the catheter tip is free within the vessel or chamber lumen (i.e., not entrapped in the chamber or vessel wall), and that all air is out of the system. (Consider other methods of air-purging when injecting a non-ionic contrast medium. There is concern that these agents can induce clot formation when mixed with blood.)

SELECTIVE ANGIOGRAPHY

Early clinical angiography was accomplished by injecting large amounts of dye into a peripheral vein (or veins) and following the course of the dye through the central circulation. This procedure is referred to as nonselective angiography. As the injection site, by means of a catheter, is brought closer to or actually into the desired chamber or vessel, the procedure is referred to as selective angiography. Four examples follow.

Pulmonary Angiography. This type of angiogram (or arteriogram) might be obtained as an isolated procedure or included in a more extensive catheterization. It is used mainly to demonstrate blood clots in the pulmonary artery branches in cases of pulmonary thromboembolism and can be useful in clarifying the nature of lung masses. An angiographic catheter (closed end, side holes), usually inserted from an antecubital vein or femoral vein, is positioned in the central pulmonary artery for the bolus dye injection with the pressure injector. The cut-film x-ray imaging system is most commonly used. Alternatively or additionally, injections are made into the pulmonary artery branches (manually or by power injector); imaging is accomplished with the cine system (cine pulmonary angiography).

Left Ventriculography. An angiogram of the left ventricle is routinely obtained as a component of a left-heart catheterization in patients with coronary artery disease, valvular heart disease, cardiomyopathy, and, often, congenital heart disease. An angiographic catheter such as a pigtail or Eppendorf type (closed end, side holes) is positioned in the chamber under pressure and fluoroscopic control. The position of the catheter tip must be adjusted so as not to induce ectopic beats by stimulation of the endocardium. An average dye bolus for an adult is 40 to 45 ml delivered by power injector in 3 or 4 sec. Because of the rapid motion, the cine technique (30 to 60 frames/sec.) is used. Single-plane projection at 30° right anterior oblique is most often employed, but bi-plane viewing, with the second projection at 60° left anterior oblique and 20 to 25° cranially angulated, adds considerable information. The left ventricle of a patient with recurrent extensive myocardial infarctions appears dilated with reduced wall motion (contractility). In a patient with mitral regurgitation, dye is seen being driven retrograde into the left atrium during systole. In an infant or child with a ventricular septal defect, a jet of dye crosses the intraventricular septum from the left ventricle to the right ventricle.

Aortography. Dye injection through an angiographic catheter with the tip located in the aortic root, just above the aortic valve, is known as an aortogram or aortic-root angiogram. Using the cine filming technique, aortic valvular insufficiency can be shown as one identifies the puffs of greater or smaller magnitude entering the left ventricle from the aorta in diastole. In severe cases, dye injected into the aortic root above the valve in essence "falls" back into the ventricle.

Chronic sacular aneurysm of the aorta is another condition well demonstrated by aortography. These aneurysms may be initially detected on the chest x-ray as a "mass." Emergency aortography is performed in cases of suspected rupture of the aorta following trauma such as a motor vehicle accident.

Finally, dissecting hematoma of the aorta (dissecting aneurysm), clinically characterized by severe chest or back pain or both, often requires aortography on an emergency basis or as soon as the clinical condition is stable. The angiographic hallmarks of aortic dissection are the appearance of contrast medium in the "false lumen," compression of the true lumen, and possibly demonstration of a linear tear in the aorta.

Coronary Angiography. Coronary angiography is one of the most important types of angiography performed today, and a more detailed discussion will therefore be given. Obstructive lesions (plaques) in the coronary arteries, which are prevalent, are responsible for the common clinical syndromes of angina and myocardial infarction.

The complete procedure almost always includes catheterization of the left ventricle for both pressure determinations and ventriculography. This is required because evaluation of structure and function of the left ventricle is an integral part of the assessment and treatment strategy of a patient with ischemic (coronary artery) heart disease.

Although the brachial artery cutdown approach developed by Sones was the first clinically reliable technique for coronary angiography, the percutaneous retrograde transfemoral (artery) technique of Judkins, with the use of an arterial sheath, has attained greater popularity (see comparison of the techniques in chapter 7).

The caliber of the catheters (French size) for coronary angiography is an important consideration. It has been customary to use 8-French catheters (and sheaths) for the percutaneous femoral technique because the torque control (turning response) of these catheters is good and manual contrast injections do not require undue effort. Smaller-sized catheters are desirable for the percutaneous technique, however, to decrease postcatheterization bleeding and hemostasis complications (usually about 10%). Until recently smaller catheters with properties similar to the larger ones have not been available. Now a number of manufacturers produce 6-French and even 5-French catheters that can perform as well as the larger ones.

This is an important development because of the advent of "outpatient" or same-day catheterization, in which the patient is not hospitalized overnight after the procedure, as has been the custom (see chapter 4). The use of a smaller catheter is thus inherently safer in cases in which a patient will be ambulating and discharged after being observed for only a few hours.

This is less of an issue with the brachial technique, with which 8-French catheters are standard. A small or spastic brachial artery may necessitate the use of a 7-French catheter. The brachial arteriotomy is directly sutured with minimal bleeding risk (see chapter 7).

When using either the Sones or Judkins technique, the left ventricle and the right and left coronary arteries, which are the first branches of the aorta as it arises from the left ventricle, are reached by a catheter passed retrograde through the arterial circulation. For the femoral technique the ventriculogram is most often obtained using a pigtail catheter (Fig. 6–3) or, less commonly, an Eppendorf-type catheter (Fig. 6–2) that has closed ends and side-holes.

With the brachial technique the Sones catheter (Fig. 6–4), which was actually developed for selective coronary angiography, can also be used for ventriculography. The physician, however, may elect to use another type of angiographic catheter (pigtail or Eppendorf) for the ventriculogram to avoid the tendency of the Sones catheter to recoil with large volume flow.

The ventriculogram is usually obtained before proceeding to selective coronary angiography. In some cases, however, the physician may wish to defer the ventriculogram until after assessing the coronary arteries, or omit it altogether. Such an approach might be considered in patients who have poor cardiac function, which increases the risk of the large bolus of contrast medium (40 to 50 ml) inordinately depressing left ventricular function, causing heart failure or shock. When ventriculography must be avoided (which is uncommon), a reasonable substitute is a good quality two-dimensional echocardiogram of the left ventricle. This "noninvasive" technique was not available until fairly recently.

After ventriculography and repeat LV-pressure determination, a Sones catheter can be withdrawn into the aortic root and directed toward selective cannulation of each coronary artery. When the femoral technique is used with an arterial sheath (usual practice at this time) it is quite simple to withdraw the pigtail or other catheter and insert one of the Judkins-type catheters, which are preshaped to allow what is usually relatively easy entry into the coronary orifice. Specific shapes are made for the left and right coronary arteries (Fig. 6–5). For selective coronary angiography with either the Judkins or Sones technique the objective is to place the tip of the catheter about 3 to 5 mm beyond the orifice of the coronary artery and obtain a series of angiograms in first one and then the other artery. Unless there is some special aspect of the patient's condition, the left coronary artery is usually studied first.

Approximately 5 to 7 ml of dye is injected manually by syringe. The angiographer will generally ask the patient to sustain a deep breath during the injection, causing the diaphragm to descend from the field of view and markedly improving the imaging of the vessels. Deeply held inspiration in some individuals causes nonspecific chest discomfort or pain, which should be differentiated from ischemic cardiac pain. This is tested by asking the patient to hold deep inspiration but without administering the dye injection. The cine system is activated during the opacification of the coronary artery for permanent recording.

Because the coronary arteries have extensive branching and because the branches have a three-dimensional configuration, multiple injections and imaging in multiple projections is mandatory for complete visualization and demonstration of obstructive lesions. Thus, right and left oblique angles are utilized for both arteries, as is a lateral projection for the left coronary artery. It is also useful to image both vessels with cranial and caudal angulation to demonstrate lesions in arteries, which are overlapped in standard views (Figs. 8–2 and 8–3).

When the catheter is inserted into the coronary artery, the arterial waveform must be closely observed by the operator, nurse, or other assistants to avoid "damping." This occurs when the catheter tip is obstructing the coronary artery and could produce dangerous ischemia. When this occurs the angiographer withdraws the catheter until a free waveform is once again present. The position of the catheter can be assessed by injecting small test doses of the dye until proper stable placement of the catheter is obtained.

The angiographer's assistants should observe the electrocardiographic monitor as much as possible, especially during the injection. When ECG lead 2 is monitored, injection into the left coronary artery can produce marked T wave inversion; injection into the right coronary artery can produce marked T wave elevation. More importantly, toward the end of the injection bradycardia commonly occurs, which is usually transient, as are the T-wave changes. Tachyarrhythmias can also occur.

One way of managing bradycardia, when severe, is to request the patient, as previously instructed, to cough hard several times. This has been called a "self-cardiac massage" and has the effect of "massaging" the angiographic dye out of the coronary circulation and restores normal heart rate. Another approach to this problem is to pretreat the patient with atropine, which may prevent bradycardia. Finally, in some circumstances the physician will insert a pacemaker wire into the right ventricle for demand pacing below a certain heart rate (e.g., 55 beats/min).

During the actual dye injection it is not possible to monitor the catheter-tip pressure, but as soon as the injection is completed the stopcock on the manifold is reset for pressure monitoring. Some hypotension occurs during and following the injection; this is partially related to the bradycardia. The pressure will normally return to baseline in a few seconds.

The injection generally causes little or no sensation. Not all the dye may actually enter the coronary artery, however, and some may reflux into the aortic root and circulate to the neck and chest regions, causing a burning sensation in the throat or upper chest. Some patients can experience angina. The assistants should frequently ask the patient if they are experiencing pain or other symptoms. The angiographer may wish to treat the patient with nitroglycerin (sublingually, intravenously, or by injecting it into the coronary artery) or possibly by administering nifedipine sublingually.

The most dreaded complication of coronary angiography is ventricular fibrillation, which occurs in about 1 of every 100 cases. This is usually seen immediately on the monitor by an alert team, even before the patient loses consciousness. (A cooperative patient can maintain consciousness by rapid hard coughing.) The defibrillator, always prepared and charged, is applied to the chest by the nurse or assistant and discharged as soon as consciousness is lost or, in any event, within 10 to 15 sec. This is almost always successful in restoring a normal rhythm, mainly because of the short duration of fibrillation. A medical decision is then made whether to continue or terminate the procedure.

On occasion a full resuscitation procedure is required, including intubation and multiple defibrillations. In rare instances, patients succumb, often after a period of electromechanical dissociation (EMD). Mortality should be less than 2 or 3 of every 1000 cases.

Coronary angiography can generally be safely and successfully performed, provided that the angiographer and the assistants are well trained and pay meticulous attention to details.

SUMMARY

Angiography is a major component of a catheterization procedure. It allows temporary visualization of a blood vessel or cardiac chamber with x-ray imaging techniques. The injected contrast medium (dye) may cause pain, vasodilation (hypotension), arrhythmia, allergic reactions, and adversely affected renal function. Modern techniques of imaging and improved dyes have made the procedure safer, less unpleasant, and more diagnostic. Virtually all veins and arteries in the body, and all of the heart chambers, can be selectively opacified for assessment of such qualities as patency, enlargement, motion (of ventricles), and abnormal flow patterns.

12

Use of Drugs in the Catheterization Laboratory

During a catheterization patients receive a wide variety of drugs. This chapter will review why and how these drugs are used and administered. No attempt will be made to discuss the drug therapy of cardiac arrest, as many other sources cover this topic.

Whenever a drug is given, it is mandatory that a record is made in the catheterization procedure flow-sheet: drug, route of administration, dose, and time.

SEDATION

Diazepam, 10 mg orally, or hydroxyzine paomate, 50 mg orally, are commonly used for precatheterization sedation. In some laboratories, diphenhydramine, 50 mg orally, is given in addition to or instead of diazepam. Meperidine and promethazine can be given as an alternative. The mixture of meperidine, promethazine, and chlopromazine effectively sedates infants and children.*

During the procedure, if patients are very restless or experiencing local pain, I.V. diazepam or morphine can be given. Attempts should first be made, however, to alleviate specific causes of pain or discomfort (such as additional local anesthetic, nitrate administration for angina, or pillow support under a sore back or ischemic lower extremities).

NITRATES

Patients experiencing angina during a procedure can be given nitroglycerine by various routes. Sublingual tablets are

---

*1.0 ml per 15 kg I.M. of a mixture containing: 1.0 ml (50 mg) meperidine, 0.5 ml (12.5 mg) each of promethazine and chlorpromazine. This is known as the "Toronto cocktail."

traditional but have the drawback that the onset of action may be delayed, as the mouth is frequently dry. A metered dose of the sublingual spray is a useful alternative.

Intravenous nitroglycerine is now available. Our laboratory routinely obtains fresh I.V. nitroglycerine solution from the hospital pharmacy in the morning. For angina, intravenous bolus doses of 25 to 75 μg can be given or, if necessary, a continuous I.V. infusion is very effective (dosages requirements above 75 to 100 μg per minute should be rare).

Nitroglycerine in any of the above forms can be used to counteract spasm (spontaneous or catheter-induced) in coronary arteries. I.V. nitroglycerine is also effective in the treatment of hypertension. The response is prompt and usually controlled.

Side effects of nitroglycerine are the well-known headache flushing and tachycardia. Excessive doses cause hypotension.

As soon as a nitrate medication is given we place a small lead-letter marker under the fluoroscope and expose a brief run of cine film. This positively identifies the point of drug administration during a sequence of (coronary) angiograms. Without this marker there can be confusion. Three different lead-letter markers are available: NGL, s.l. (sublingual); NGL, i.v. (intravenous); and NGL, i.c. (intracoronary). The letters are taped to a tongue blade.

ANTICOAGULANTS AND PROTOMINE

With some increased risk of bleeding, urgent catheterization, preferably by cutdown, can be performed when the prothrombin time (PT) is elevated up to 18 sec. (control: 11 to 12 sec.) in patients being treated with anticoagulants (coumarin derivatives). The PT should be 15 sec. or less. For elective catheterizations it is not advisable to try to lower the PT rapidly with parenteral vitamin K; it is preferable to let the PT drift down slowly and spontaneously. In an emergency in which the PT is greater than 20 sec., fresh frozen plasma and vitamin K can be given.

In a patient with a prosthetic heart valve, it might be dangerous to discontinue anticoagulant therapy (warfarin sodium), particularly if the patient has experienced thromboembolism. In such a case I.V. heparin can be initiated, after which the oral anticoagulant is discontinued. The catheterization is delayed until the PT decreases to less than 14 to 15 sec. Finally, I.V. heparin is withheld 4 hours before beginning the procedure, a period short enough to avoid thrombus development on a prosthetic valve. Chronic aspirin therapy is not considered a contraindication to catheterization.

Heparin is usually administered to patients undergoing left-heart or arterial procedures. Radiologists performing peripheral angiography may omit the use of heparin. This can be given intravenously into the distal brachial artery after direct exposure (cutdown) or into the aorta after catheter insertion. The standard dose is 5000 I.U. (For angioplasty, 10,000 I.U. is preferred.) Only vials with 1000 I.U./ml are stocked in the catheterization laboratory to avoid inadvertant administration of an excessive dose.

When a percutaneous procedure is completed many cardiologists will "reverse" or "neutralize" the heparin, at least partially, through the administration of protamine sulfate intravenously to reduce puncture-site bleeding. Full reversal requires approximately 1 mg protamine for every 100 I.U. of heparin (i.e., 50 mg for the usual 5000-IU dose of heparin. In our laboratory we usually administer 25 to 35 mg of protamine I.V. slowly (over 4 to 5 min.) to prevent hypotension, just before the catheter or sheath removal, particularly if the procedure has been of short duration. Protamine is not used after brachial artery cutdown procedures or after balloon angioplasty. The heparin/protamine combination is effective in reducing both thrombotic and bleeding complications. In diabetic patients being treated with NPH (neutral *protamine* Hagedorn) insulin, there have been reports of allergic-type reactions, which are manifested by hypotension, bronchospasm, pulmonary hypertension, and death (in 1 to 2 patients per 10,000), following the administration of protamine at the end of a procedure for heparin neutralization. There is no reason to abandon the use of protamine in these patients, but the staff should be alert to the possibility of a reaction and ready to undertake treatment as the physician indicates. This would include administration of epinephrine, I.V. fluids, pressor agents, steroids, H1 and H2 antihistamines, and intubation for laryngospasm—all standard for treatment of drug reactions.

ATROPINE

Atropine sulfate, administered intravenously, in doses from 0.5 mg to 2.0 mg, is used primarily to combat excessive bradycardia. Patients frequently demonstrate bradycardia at the beginning of the procedure or respond to the pain of local anesthetization (or its anticipation) with vagal mediated bradycardia. Another common cause for bradycardia is prior treatment with beta blockers or calcium entry blockers (e.g., diltiazem).

Some cardiologists use atropine as needed to treat bradycardia; others use it routinely. I generally administer the drug if the pulse rate is less than 70 to 75 beats/min, since I have observed that with higher heart rates profound or symptomatic bradycardia rarely occurs, even during coronary angiography. However, atropine can easily be given at any time during the procedure, with prompt onset of action. For example, if a coronary contrast injection produces a heart rate of less than 50 beats/min for more than a few seconds (a more frequent occurrence after dye injection of the right than the left coronary artery), atropine is given and in 1 to 2 min. subsequent injections can be made, usually without the bradycardia. In the future, as improved contrast media are more widely used, bradycardia may be less common.

The main side effect of atropine, dry mouth, is alleviated by having the patient suck on a moistened sponge. Excessive dosing of atropine is to be avoided because sinus tachycardia can also be harmful.

BETA BLOCKERS

Many patients who have been treated chronically with a beta blocker arrive at the catheterization laboratory with bradycardia (see under Atropine). During the procedure intravenous beta blocker can be used to treat supraventricular tachycardia, slow the rapid ventricular response in atrial fibrillation, or even slow the rate of sinus tachycardia when the latter is "inappropriate" (excessive emotional reaction). Typical doses would be: propranolol, 2.5 to 5 mg I.V. and metoprolol, 5 to 15 mg I.V. Esmolol, recently available, has a very rapid onset and short half-life. A bolus dose of 0.5 mg/kg, I.V. in 1 min. followed by a maintenance infusion of 50 μg/kg/min. is standard.

For severe or uncontrolled hypertension, 20 to 40 mg I.V. bolus doses of labetalol are useful. Maintenance doses of 1 or 2 mg/min. of labetalol can be used after or instead of the bolus.

The main side effects of beta blockade, aside from excessive bradycardia, are bronchospasm and cardiac functional depression.

CALCIUM CHANNEL BLOCKERS

These relatively newly available drugs can be useful. Verapamil, 5-to 10-mg I.V. bolus, is effective in the treatment of supraventricular tachycardia. Nifedipine, 10 mg sublingual, is used for vasospastic angina. Nifedipine can also be used for hypertension. The best way to administer this drug for rapid action is to have the patient bite the capsule and then swallow capsule and contents.

Hypotension and excess bradycardia (verapamil) are the main side effects of these drugs. Many new types of calcium channel blockers are being developed.

ANTIARRHYTHMICS

For frequent premature ventricular beats or ventricular tachycardia, lidocaine is the main drug in use, 1 to 2 boluses, 75 mg and 50 mg each, followed by a maintenance dose of at least 2 mg/min. or 3 to 5 mg/min. in more serious situations. Procainamide is an alternative when lidocaine is ineffective. Bretylium tosylate, 5 mg/Kg I.V. bolus, is also useful in the treatment of ventricular tachycardia or fibrillation.

PRESSOR AGENTS

Hypotension can occur because of acute depression of cardiac function, vasodilation (drug reaction), or hypovolemia. The latter is encountered in patients who are dehydrated and especially after diuretic treatment. Rapid infusion of physiologic saline intravenously (or rapid intraortic infusions of 20-ml boluses) can reverse hypovolemia.

Dopamine, in I.V. dosages of 5 to 20 μg/kg/min. is the routine treatment for nonhypovolemic hypotension.

DIURETICS

When acute pulmonary congestion occurs during catheterization, standard intravenous furosamide, 40 to 80-mg bolus, is commonly used. Other drugs with similar action are bumetadine and ethacrynic acid. The decongestive effect can occur before diuresis because of venous pooling.

ERGONOVINE

Ergonovine maleate is used to demonstrate sensitivity of the coronary arteries to spasm. There are various protocols for administration. I use I.V. doses of 50, 100, and 150 μg separated by 5 to 8 min. After each dose, blood pressure, pulse, and ECG are observed, and the patient is assessed for symptoms (angina, headache). Coronary angiograms are also obtained after each dose. With high-enough doses, spasm can be induced in virtually all coronary arteries. Spasm is usually easy to reverse with sublingual or I.V. nitroglycerine. At times intracoronary nitroglycerine has been required.

As described in the section on nitroglycerine administration, a lead-letter marker is exposed on the cine film after every dose (e.g., ERGO, 100 μg).

DIGOXIN

This drug was more frequently used to treat supraventricular arrhythmia before the development of drugs such as beta blockers or calcium channel blockers. It is now rarely used in the cath lab.

TREATMENT OF CONTRAST MEDIA (DYE) REACTIONS

The immediate responses to contrast media (aside from expected flushing and headache, transient hypotension, and cardiac depression) that signify an allergic response include urticaria and itching, bronchospasm, (rarely) laryngospasm and edema, prolonged hypotension, and bradycardia. In mild cases (urticaria) I.M. or I.V. diphenyhydramine hydrochloride 25 to 50 mg is used. For mild to moderate bronchospasm any of the sympaticomimetic amine inhalors (isoproterenol, terbutaline) can be used, along with I.V. epinephrine 1.0 ml of 1:10,000 dilution. When hypotension and bradycardia occur, depending on severity, treatment can include rapid infusion of I.V. fluid, atropine 2.0 μg I.V., dopamine, 10 to 20 μg/kg/min, and I.V. hydrocortisone 100 to 500 mg (30 sec. to 10 min.). Intubation is necessary for laryngospasm.

DRUG SUPPLIES

All of the drugs mentioned above should be stocked in the cath lab.

The usual I.V. solutions, such as physiologic saline, 0.45 N saline, and 5 and 10% dextrose in water, are standard items. Intravenous pumps are now in routine use.

A "Crash Cart" containing drugs and equipment for resuscitation is ordinarily available in most laboratories.

A comprehensive drug list should include the following:

Aminophyllin
Atropine sulfate
Bretylium tosylate
Calcium chloride
Calcium gluconate
Chlorpromazine
Diazepam (p.o, i.v.)
Digoxin (p.o., i.v.)
Diltiazem
Diphenlhydramine
Dobutamine
Dopamine
Edrophonium
Ergonovine maleate
Epinephrine
Esmolol
Furosemide
Haloperidol (p.o., i.v.)
Heparin

Hydrocortisone
Hydroxyzine (p.o., i.v.)
Labetalol (i.v.)
Lidocaine
Magnesium sulfate
Meperidine
Metaraminol
Metoprolol (p.o., i.v.)
Morphine sulfate
Nifedipine
Nitroglycerine (s.l., i.v.)
Phentolamine
Phenytoin (p.o., i.v.)
Potassium chloride
Procainamide
Prostigmine
Protamine
Sodium-nitroprusside
Verapamil (p.o., i.v.)

Miscellaneous items:
Bacitracin ointment
Povidone-iodine
Topical thrombin

13

Therapeutic or Interventional Catheterization: Angioplasty

Cardiovascular catheterization was developed primarily as a diagnostic tool. However, with technical advances and experience, it became apparent that the catheter could also be used therapeutically. Thus, there has been increasing interest in "interventional" catheterization, that is, a catheter technique used to administer medication or perform surgical manipulation. Although the general public is now aware of transluminal angioplasty, using a balloon on the end of a catheter to dilate a stenotic coronary artery as an alternative to coronary bypass surgery, there are other useful "interventions" that can be performed with a catheter. This chapter will describe varieties of angioplasty; chapter 14 will review some of the other techniques.

HISTORIC PERSPECTIVES

In 1963, the late Dr. Charles T. Dotter, a West Coast radiologist, originated the idea that a catheter could be used to dilate an artery obstructed by atherosclerotic plaque or thrombus. In obtaining a routine angiogram, he threaded a catheter by the usual retrograde percutaneous technique from the right femoral artery into the abdominal aorta. After studying the x-ray films, Dotter realized that the catheter had passed through a *totally occluded iliac artery* that was filled (presumably) with relatively soft thrombus throughout its length. Dotter then reasoned that if a catheter could be threaded through a blocked vessel inadvertently, deliberate passage, *for therapeutic purposes* (i.e., to enlarge the lumen), could also be accomplished. His first case (reported in 1964 with Judkins) was an elderly patient with gangrene of the foot caused by stenosis of the popliteal artery. Dotter inserted a guidewire antegrade from the femoral artery and passed the flexible tip of the wire across the stenosis. The guidewire was then used to track a series of successively larger catheters across the stenosis until it was fully dilated. These

dilating catheters functioned as a type of bougie. He reported that
". . . the prompt return of circulation to her foot and the ensuing
reversal of her gangrene made little inroads on the skepticism of
colleagues. . . ."

Following this important clinical advance, interest in nonsurgical dilation of arteries, known as transluminal angioplasty
("PTA" when the dilating catheter is inserted percutaneously,
"PTCA" when the coronary arteries are being dilated), centered in
Europe and was mainly ignored in the United States. The late Dr.
A. Grüntzig, working in Zurich, Switzerland, developed the
modern balloon catheter, which stimulated a renewed interest in
angioplasty. This technique was simpler, effective, and had a
lower complication rate than the earlier, cruder approaches.

Initially the main application of balloon angioplasty was in
the area of peripheral vascular disease, particularly of the lower
extremities. Later, Grüntzig miniaturized the system so it could
be used in the treatment of coronary artery disease.

PTA—BALLOON ANGIOPLASTY FOR PERIPHERAL VASCULAR DISEASE

Atherosclerotic obstruction of the arteries supplying the
lower extremities is common in middle-aged and elderly people
and may be particularly severe in diabetics. The classic symptom
is intermittent claudication. Characteristically, patients are comfortable at rest but develop calf pain or thigh and hip pain
(depending upon location of the arterial blockage) with walking.
The blood flow to the leg is adequate at rest but the narrowed
vessel does not supply enough blood to the muscles during the
increased demand of exercise. The inadequate blood flow (ischemia) results in pain. The condition may be very mild in some
patients but can limit walking to less than 100 to 200 ft in others.
Eventually blood flow may decrease further, resulting in pain at
rest and possibly tissue breakdown (gangrene). Patients with
such symptoms ordinarily undergo diagnostic angiography to
evaluate the lower aorta and arterial blood supply to both legs.
When vascular narrowings are demonstrated the decision to
proceed with angioplasty is best made along with the vascular
surgeon. Successful angioplasty has the obvious advantage of
avoiding formal surgery, particularly in older and debilitated
patients, and can be repeated if necessary.

The patient is prepared for angioplasty in a similar manner
as for a routine transfemoral artery catheterization. Aspirin, an
antithrombotic agent, is often given before the procedure. Standard local anesthesia is used. If the lesion to be dilated is in the
iliac artery, the puncture needle is inserted retrograde (in the

direction of the iliac artery) and antegrade if the lesion is located in the superficial femoral or popliteal arteries. Straight or J guidewires are inserted through the needle and manipulated carefully through and beyond the stenotic area, after which the needle is withdrawn. To facilitate subsequent catheter insertion, a dilator (7 or 8 French) is first passed over the guidewire into the blood vessel and then removed. The balloon catheter (balloon deflated) can then be tracked over the wire into the artery. The use of a vascular sheath is also possible.

The balloon catheter has two lumens. The central lumen allows insertion over the guidewire, pressure measurements, and contrast medium injection. The second lumen is used for balloon inflation. A typical catheter would have a 7-French shaft and a balloon 2 cm in length near the tip, with an inflated diameter of 2 to 8 mm. The large size is selected for a large vessel such as the iliac artery, a 4-mm balloon is standard for femoral artery dilations, and the smaller sizes are used for small branches below the knee. The balloons are generally made of polyethylene and can be inflated up to 6 to 8 atmospheres. Balloon inflation, using dilute contrast medium (which makes the balloon visible on fluoroscopy) is facilitated by use of a mechanical syringe with an in-line pressure gauge, connected by a short length of pressure tubing to the balloon port of the catheter. Metallic markers allow easy fluoroscopic location of the balloon in the absence of contrast (i.e., when the balloon is deflated). During insertion into the artery or passage through a tight stenosis, negative pressure is applied to the balloon to make its profile as small as possible. After insertion of the catheter it is necesesary to inject dye (manually) into the vessel for exact localization of the stenotic lesion(s) intended for dilation. This is aided by the use of a long, radiopaque ruler placed externally along the side of the patient's leg or pelvis. Replay from the VCR then shows the lesion at a particular location on the ruler. The catheter is advanced over the guidewire so as to position the balloon exactly across the stenotic area.

Multiple inflations are generally used (with pressures up to manufacturers' specifications and maintained for 30 to 60 sec. or longer, usually without much, if any, discomfort or pain). After balloon deflation, test injections of contrast media, as seen on fluoroscopy (stored for replay on the VCR), enable the operator to assess the results. It is also possible to measure intra-arterial pressure, with the expectation that the pressure drop, typically noted in the artery beyond the stenosis, decreases or disappears.

The mechanism of balloon angioplasty is not completely understood; the response may not be the same from patient to patient since the underlying pathology of the stenotic plaque varies (Fig. 13–1). Dilation results from compression and remod-

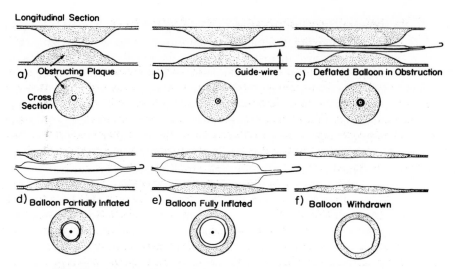

Fig. 13—1. *Schematic principles of angioplasty. A. Artery with local athero-sclerotic obstruction. B. Guidewire advanced across lesion. C. Balloon catheter tracked over guidewire (balloon deflated). D. Partial balloon inflation. The atherosclerotic plaque is split, compressed, and redistributed longitudinally, and the vessel is stretched. E. Full balloon dilation. F. Balloon catheter and guidewire withdrawn.*

eling of the plaque, stretching of the entire vessel, longitudinal fissuring of the plaque, etc. This "controlled injury" (Grüntzig), which is irregular and ragged as a pathology specimen or when observed in vivo with an angioscope (catheter for direct intravascular visualization), may later undergo a smoothing and healing process with the development of a new intimal lining.

In properly selected cases the initial success rate of dilation and improvement in flow can be as high as 90 to 95%. Patency can be expected in about 80% of cases after a year, but restenosis will eventually recur in most cases after a long-enough period of time. The best long-term results are with the larger iliac arteries, as opposed to the smaller vessels at or below the knee. Balloon angioplasty must be considered palliative because the underlying disease process is not altered. Restenosis may be retarded by strict control of blood lipid levels.

The major risks of the procedure are injury to the artery at the site of entry and groin hematoma. Vascular surgery may be needed to manage such problems.

Renal artery angioplasty is accomplished essentially as explained above and is undertaken in cases of renal hypertension and, less commonly, for renal insufficiency.

PTCA—BALLOON ANGIOPLASTY OF THE CORONARY ARTERIES

With miniaturization and some modification, Grüntzig adopted the balloon angioplasty principle, developed initially for peripheral vascular disease, for dilation of stenosed coronary arteries. This important advance in the treatment of coronary disease provided an alternative to the only other means of direct myocardial revascularization: coronary artery bypass graft surgery (open-heart surgery).

When the atherosclerotic plaque reduces the coronary arterial lumen area by about 70%, flow can remain adequate with the patient at rest. With activity, however, flow does not increase to meet the increased demands required of the heart muscle. Thus, patients can experience exertional chest pain, or angina (cardiac ischemia), during activity or emotional stress. The pain disappears with rest. Medication may ameliorate the symptoms. Diagnostic coronary angiography in these patients delineates the location and degree of the blockages, which are often multiple (i.e., in all three major coronary branches). The stenotic process may affect an artery in a local segment or may be present throughout the length of the vessel. The first patients selected for angioplasty were those with single segmental obstructions fairly close to the origin of the branch. With improved techniques multivessel angioplasty of lesser accessible lesions became possible.

The most important drawback to PTCA is that it can cause a partially stenosed artery to become totally occluded, which can result in rapid onset of ischemic pain, hemodynamic deterioration, or arrhythmia, possibly requiring emergency coronary bypass surgery. Such an outcome occurs in only about 5% of cases; nevertheless, to avoid unnecessary delay in instituting emergency surgery, it is usual, when scheduling a patient for PTCA, to also make arrangements with the cardiac surgeon and the operating room for standby availability. Thus, a patient with coronary disease who is a candidate for treatment with PTCA would otherwise be considered for bypass surgery. On the other hand, if PTCA fails but does not lead to acute clinical deterioration, bypass surgery can be undertaken electively if appropriate. Clearly, the patient must be fully informed about these issues. Support staff in the laboratory also must be familiar with them to help the patients through the procedure and assist the medical staff in managing problems.

Balloon angioplasty was originally developed using the percutaneous transfemoral modified Seldinger technique. Although this approach continues to be the most commonly utilized, similar results can be achieved using the direct cutdown retrograde brachial artery technique. In either case, the main components of the system are a guiding catheter, a balloon dilating catheter (which passes through the guiding catheter), and a special "steerable" guidewire for tracking the balloon catheter through the stenosed coronary artery. A description of the "over-the-wire" technique follows (Fig. 13–2).

The general preparation of the patient is similar to that required for a diagnostic study. Most patients are treated with aspirin (an antiplatelet-aggregation agent) for 48 hours before the procedure. Some physicians also pretreat patients with the antiplatelet agent dipyridamole and may infuse low-molecular-weight dextran at the start of the procedure (an antithrombotic).

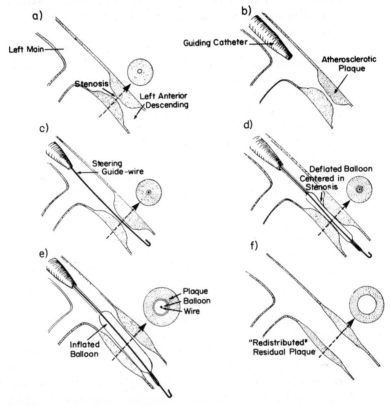

Fig. 13–2. Diagrams illustrating coronary balloon angioplasty (PTCA) of the proximal left anterior descending branch. Cross-sections are shown throughout the stenotic segment. A. Stenosis (the inner silhouette would be demonstrated angiographically. B. Guiding catheter in orifice of the left main branch. C. Balloon catheter advanced to opening of the guiding catheter and steerable guidewire advanced across the lesion. D. Balloon catheter (balloon deflated) advanced over the guidewire and centered in the stenotic segment. E. Balloon inflated, splitting, compressing, and "redistributing" the atherosclerotic plaque and stretching the arterial segment. F. After balloon deflation and withdrawal of the balloon catheter and wire, there is a small degree of residual stenosis

A 10-mg dose of nifedipine is often administered along with a continuous IV infusion of nitroglycerin, 10μg / min, which both inhibit coronary artery spasm.

A nurse or technician, after training, is often assigned to the important task of preparing the balloon catheter and the pressure gauge/syringe assembly. Standard balloon catheters (which cost in excess of $600) have a 4.3-French shaft, and inflated balloon diameters between 2 and 4 mm. Recent technologic advances have produced balloon catheters that track down the coronary arteries and cross stenoses more easily. This has been achieved by reducing the bulk, or "profile," of the balloon by replacing polyethylene with PET (polyethylene teraphthalate) and increasing the lubricity of the balloon surface with silicone. Also available now are more miniaturized balloon catheters with shafts 3.7 French or smaller.

Metallic markers on the shaft near the balloon allow for its fluoroscopic localization. The proximal end of the catheter has a channel marked "balloon" that is used for inflation and deflation. The central catheter channel opens at the tip. This can be used for pressure measurement and contrast injection, but is primarily for the "steerable" guidewire, which is very thin and flexible ("floppy" tip), 0.14 to 0.18 in. in diameter.

A "Y" connector is attached to the hub of the central lumen of the balloon catheter. One arm of the Y is attached by tubing to a standard manifold, and the other is used for passing the steerable wire through the balloon catheter to its tip. A gasket in the hub of the Y connector prevents blood leakage around the inserted wire.

Modern pressure gauge/syringes are simple mechanical devices, easy to fill with dilute contrast media and purge of air. Disposable units are now available. With an ordinary syringe, dilute contrast medium is also injected into the balloon channel of the dilating catheter to purge air. Air bubbles must be avoided when the pressure gauge/syringe is attached with a length of semi-rigid tubing to the balloon channel.

With many patients the operator begins the procedure with percutaneous insertion, from the femoral vein, of a temporary pacemaker catheter for positioning in the right heart. A Myler catheter used for this purpose can pace the RV and monitor pulmonary pressure or provide an additional IV access line. The pacing catheter is connected to a pacemaker, pacing is tested, and the pacemaker is set at a standby (demand) rate of 50 to 55 beats/min. This prevents profound bradycardia.

An arterial sheath is then placed in the femoral artery by percutaneous technique. The sheath is slightly different from the one used for routine diagnostic purposes; it has a two-stage dilator and is longer (23 cm compared to 11 cm). 10,000 IU heparin is administered intravenously. The guiding catheter is then inserted with the aid of a (large) 0.63 in. J guidewire and advanced to the aortic root, when the wire is removed.

The guiding catheter is similar to a standard ("diagnostic") angiographic catheter (Judkins) except that it has a thinner wall and a Teflon lining, which facilitates the passage of the balloon angioplasty catheter. The shaft is also firmer to allow solid "seating" in the coronary artery orifice. Guiding catheters are also available with tip shapes that are different from the usual Judkins left or right (Amplatz, Williams, El-Gamal, Arani). Such catheters can be used to obtain even firmer seating of the tip in the coronary orifice. This may be necessary when the particular anatomy of a patient (aortic root size, take-off angle of the coronary) causes the Judkins-shaped guiding catheters to retract or back out from the coronary orifice as the balloon catheter or wire is being advanced, making this maneuver difficult or impossible.

The guiding catheter is manipulated into the left or right coronary orifice (left- or right-shaped guiding catheter), and a standard coronary angiogram is obtained. This allows confirmation and location of the previously established stenosis. Some internal structure, such as the shaft of the right-heart catheter or an externally placed metallic instrument (surgical clamp), "marks" the point in the vessel designated for dilatation. Also helpful is a video freeze-frame or cine loop of the coronary angiogram and the stenosis.

Next, a special Y connector is attached to the guiding catheter hub. One arm is connected to the standard manifold for flushing, contrast medium injection, and pressure recording. The other arm allows insertion of the balloon catheter/steering wire assembly into the guiding catheter. A Touhy-Borst adapter on the arm of the Y connector is adjusted to permit balloon catheter movement but prevent blood leakage. The steering wire is retained just inside the balloon catheter tip; the balloon is maintained under negative pressure with the pressure gauge/syringe to reduce its "profile."

The operator advances the balloon catheter to the tip of the guide catheter. If pressures are recorded they should be the same from both catheters. Fluoroscopy is used as the flexible steering wire is then advanced beyond the balloon catheter tip and, by careful manipulation, tracked through the stenosis. The balloon catheter can now be advanced along the wire so that the center of the balloon, its metallic markers identified fluoroscopically, is in the stenotic arterial segment.

The pressure gauge/syringe device is used to inflate the balloon (according to the manufacturers' specifications) from 5 to 12 atmospheres. The expansion of the balloon (with contrast medium) is observed fluoroscopically. Inflation is maintained from 10 to 60 seconds (or longer). It is crucial to observe the patient for chest pain (angina), which is not uncommon, and to watch monitors for arrhythmia and hypotension.

After balloon deflation, an assessment of the effects of dilation is made by contrast injections through the guiding catheter or balloon catheter and, in some cases, by showing a trend towards equalization of pressures recorded proximal and distal to the lesion. Multiple balloon inflations are usually required to obtain acceptable results.

If a decrease in the stenosis cannot be accomplished the physician will at least make sure that a total blockage has not developed. Such an outcome, if not due to spasm that can be relieved with intracoronary nitroglycerine injection, is usually accompanied by ischemic chest pain, S-T segment shifts, hypotension, etc. Emergency bypass surgery is required, with possible prior insertion of an intra-aortic balloon pump for circulatory support. In experienced laboratories the initial success rate for achieving significant dilatation is about 90%. Emergency surgery may be required in about 5% of cases. Other complications include bleeding at the entrance site of the catheter, life-threatening arrhythmia, stroke, and steering-wire breakage with fragments in the coronary artery requiring surgical removal.

The stable patient then returns to the CCU for about 24 hours. The arterial and venous sheaths remain in place with slow infusion to maintain patency. Intravenous heparin is administered (PTT 2.5 × control) for 24 hours. The patient is observed for signs of ischemia, i.e., recurrent angina, arrhythmia, hypotension, and S-T segment shifts on the ECG and bleeding (sheath site, GI tract, etc.). Ischemic symptoms may require an angiographic reevaluation, which can be quickly accomplished using the arterial sheath.

In routine cases the sheaths are removed after the PTT normalizes; about 6 hours later the patient can ambulate. No definitive drug therapy following PTCA has been developed. Protocols have included aspirin, dipydriamole, and calcium channel blockers.

Presently, the major drawback of PTCA is the restenosis rate of about 25%. A number of patients have undergone a second procedure with approximately the same results. Diminishing returns generally makes bypass a better alternative than a third PTCA.

Finally, PTCA has been performed in a setting of acute myocardial infarction, with or without concommitant thrombolytic therapy. The aim here is to promptly (within 3 to 4 hours) restore perfusion to recently infarcted myocardium. After thrombolytic therapy has lysed a thrombus in the coronary artery, PTCA serves to dilate the underlying stenosis (which is frequently present). An efficient laboratory is required to undertake such procedures: all personnel must be fully ready to set up the equipment quickly and monitor and manage the acutely ill patient. Recent data indicate that it is preferable to delay angiography or angioplasty or both for at least several days postinfarction when the patient is stable.

Essentially the same equipment and approach can be used for dilating stenosis in vein grafts that extend from the aorta to points beyond blockages in coronary arteries. Slightly different forms of guiding catheters are used for this purpose.

Another recent modification replaces the steerable guidewire with a fixed extension on the tip of the catheter, in front of the balloon (Fig. 13–3). This obviates the need for the central lumen (used for the steerable guidewire in the usual "over-the-wire" angioplasty balloon catheter) and thus permits the construction of a catheter shaft (actually a hollow flexible wire) of very small diameter (1.7 French compared to the standard 4.3 French). Used in conjunction with a standard 8-French guiding catheter, this thin "balloon on a wire" reduces internal resistance in the guiding catheter, which makes it much easier to inject contrast through the guiding catheter to assess the progress of the angioplasty procedure. Another advantage is that *two* of these devices can be inserted through the same guiding catheter (for the two-balloon angioplasty technique).

Finally some patients undergoing "invasive" procedures such as angioplasty are in a precarious state due to such conditions as recent infarction or unstable angina. A new technique uses an extracorporeal pump oxygenator (ECPO) to provide temporary hemodynamic support during the procedure. Large-bore (18 to 20 French) cannulae are inserted, percutaneously or by cutdown, into the femoral artery and vein. Blood flows from the vein into the device, is oxygenated, and is pumped back into the artery. Functionally, this provides partial cardiopulmonary bypass. Flow rates of 4 to 5 l/min. have been achieved, thereby taking over a large part of the circulation from the heart. The device can function even during cardiac arrest. Drawbacks to the technique

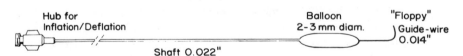

Hub for Inflation/Deflation   Shaft 0.022"   Balloon 2-3 mm diam.   "Floppy" Guide-wire 0.014"

Fig. 13–3. Diagram of "balloon" on a wire device. The balloon material (PET—polyethylene teraphthalate) is extremely thin, so the balloon presents a very narrow profile around a thin, flexible core wire (not shown). Compared with the standard "over-the-wire" balloon angioplasty catheter, this device has no lumen for contrast injection or pressure measurements, a sacrifice made to achieve simpler technique and easier passage through tight stenoses.

include injury to blood vessels, infection, and hemolysis. The ultimate utility of the technique is uncertain.

A more standard circulatory support device is the intra-aortic balloon pump (IABP), which usually can be inserted into the femoral artery percutaneously for angioplasty in an unstable patient. Unlike the ECPO, the IABP requires intrinsic cardiac activity for effective function.

EXPERIMENTAL ANGIOPLASTY TECHNIQUES

Although Grüntzig's balloon angioplasty technique represents a major breakthrough in the nonsurgical approach to reestablishing the flow through a narrowed blood vessel, it cannot be considered a definitive treatment since offending atherosclerotic plaque is not removed from the artery. An intense effort is being made to devise techniques that actually remove the blockage.

Lasers. Laser energy delivered by a fiberoptic catheter can vaporize plaque. A variety of wavelengths produced by different devices have been tried both experimentally and, to a limited degree, in humans. The work has been done mainly by surgeons in the operating room in directly exposed peripheral arteries and coronary arteries. The major problem is that it has been difficult to limit the vaporization to plaque and avoid damage or perforation of the arterial wall.

A modification of the direct lasing technique is the "hot-tip" technique, whereby laser energy carried by optic fibers packaged in a catheter is used to heat a sapphire or metal tip. This tip then burns a channel through a blocking atherosclerotic plaque. An electric "hot-tip" catheter for burning through atheromatous plaques is also undergoing evaluation.

Finally, a new approach combines balloon angioplasty and a laser. While the balloon is inflated, a laser fiber inside the balloon heats the surrounding vessel wall to about 95° C. After balloon deflation, the "heat-set" arterial wall is much less likely to collapse. It is hoped that the long term patency rate will be better.

Rotating Drill. An entirely different approach is the rotating drill-type catheter. In this technique the catheter tip is fitted with a metallic rotating head (and high-pressure fluid flush system) that spins at rates up to 10,000 RPM. This device has lysed stenosing plaques experimentally and in some patients. Perforations have occurred, which is a major drawback.

This crude "drill" has been modified by developing a drill tip that can be tracked over a guidewire previously inserted through a stenosis. The rotating head is actually a small ceramic bead studded with diamond chips. It pulverizes plaque into microscopic particles that pass through the myocardial microcirculation. This system may have less of a tendency to perforate the vessel.

Atherectomy Catheter. Finally, an atherectomy catheter has been used to remove plaque. In this system the tip of the catheter is a short tube with a slot in one side. When inflated, a balloon on the opposite side presses the slotted segment against the plaque, some of which enters the tube. A rotating blade is then advanced, slicing off the plaque expressed into the tube. The plaque is retained in the tip of the catheter and removed with catheter withdrawal.

These techniques should be considered developmental; experience with them is limited. However, it is reasonable to expect refinements and improvements in the future. Thus, increasing numbers of patients will undergo interventional procedures.

14

Therapeutic or Interventional Catheterization: Other Techniques

In this chapter we will review other important techniques that utilize a catheter to deliver medication or perform surgical manipulation or treatment.

USING THE CATHETER TO INSTILL MEDICATION

For a variety of indications different medications can be infused with a catheter. With the tip selectively positioned in a specific artery, relatively high concentrations of drugs can be targeted to an organ or vascular region, allowing the use of lower overall doses. One of the most important applications of this technique is for lysis of coronary and peripheral artery thrombi.

It has been known for more than 30 years that certain agents, injected into the blood, can induce lysis of intravascular thrombi or clots. Streptokinase (SK), a bacterial enzyme, converts plasminogen, a natural factor present in the blood, into plasmin, which is an active enzyme capable of breaking down fibrin, a major component of the blood clot. An early clinical use of SK, administered intravenously, was for the lysis of clots located in the pulmonary arteries.

Although thrombus formation in coronary arteries has been known to be associated with myocardial infarction, the causative role of thrombus has only recently been delineated and understood. This insight resulted from the practice of obtaining coronary angiograms in patients early after myocardial infarction. It was later demonstrated that a relatively small dose of streptokinase, infused directly by catheter into the right or left coronary, could lyse a thrombus situated downstream with subsequent restoration of blood flow. If this can be accomplished quickly (within 6 hours, preferably within 4 hours) after inception of the infarct, damage to the myocardium can be limited.

To accomplish this there must be prompt clinical recognition of the condition, which means that the patient must arrive

97

quickly at the hospital and the diagnosis must be readily apparent. The patient then has to be rapidly transported to a laboratory that has personnel and equipment ready to function in minutes. The procedure is carried out in the usual manner for standard catheterization and coronary angiogram. The laboratory staff, in addition to being promptly mobilized, must be especially alert and observant of the patient, who is in a precarious state and is prone to develop arrhythmia, heart failure, conduction disturbances, etc. Blood is withdrawn for baseline testing, including PT, PTT, fibrinogen, prothrombin time, and thrombin time.

After the physician identifies the "culprit" artery, i.e., the right or left coronary artery containing the thrombus, the catheter tip is maintained in the coronary artery and streptokinase (3000 to 5000 IU/min) is infused (a relatively low dose). At intervals of 10 to 15 min. test angiograms are made to determine if clot lysis has occurred. Infusion is continued until the clot lyses or up to a maximum dose of about 600,000 IU SK are given. Lysis can be expected in 30 to 60 min. in about 75% of cases. This is associated clinically with a decrease in S-T segment elevation, a decrease in ischemic pain and possibly the appearance of "reperfusion" arrhythmia (ventricular ectopic beats occurring transiently).

Urokinase, a naturally occurring and therefore nonantigenic human enzyme with plasminogen-activating properties, can also be used for intracoronary administration with essentially the same results. With either SK or UK, despite the advantages of using a relatively low dose, systemic effects still occur with resultant reduction of fibrinogen, increasing thrombin time, and other conditions that can manifest in significant clinical bleeding (e.g., skin, GI tract, and intracerebral). Because of this, thrombolytic therapy is not used in patients with active bleeding, within 2 months of a stroke, within 10 days of major surgery, after recent serious trauma, or during pregnancy.

Although there was considerable enthusiasm for this procedure initially and impressive results, the difficult logistics and inherent time delays stimulated interest in the use of thrombolytic agents administered intravenously, the approach now more commonly used.

A novel application of UK, using a catheterization technique, is to lyse clots in aortocoronary vein grafts. Blockage of flow through the grafts may result in myocardial ischemia with clinical manifestations of angina. The procedure is carried out electively and entails inserting a catheter, introduced percutaneously from the femoral artery, into the origin of the graft and infusing a low concentration of UK (thereby reducing side effects) for up to 72 hours. The patient is in the catheterization laboratory only during catheter insertion and for test angiograms to assess the progress of the treatment.

Thrombolytic agents delivered by catheter are also used in cases of thrombus in peripheral arteries, such as the femoral or popliteal, in a manner similar to that used for lysis of coronary artery clots.

Catheter delivery of medication to specific sites or organs has been used in a few other miscellaneous conditions, such as cancer chemotherapeutic agents infused into the hepatic artery or adrenal arteries for treatment of cancer in these organs and vasopressen infusion into the superior mesenteric artery to reduce GI tract bleeding, etc.

PROCEDURES IN CONGENITAL HEART DISEASE

Balloon Atrial Septostomy. Infants born with some congenital heart anomalies are known as "blue babies" because venous (dark) blood reaches the arterial circulation. This is also often associated with inadequate blood flow through the lungs, resulting in inadequate blood oxygenation. The classic abnormality is transposition of the great vessels, whereby the aorta exits from the right ventricle and therefore circulates venous blood to the systemic circulation, and the pulmonary artery exits from the left ventricle and carries oxygenated blood back to the lungs. For there to be any possibility of survival after birth some blood shunting between the two anatomically separate circulations must occur, usually through the ductus arteriosus. Early mortality is high in these infants without some palliative operative procedure. However, thoracotomy and cardiac surgery also carries a high operative risk.

In 1966, the late Dr. William Rashkind reported a technique that used a balloon catheter to treat these tiny patients. By standard catheterization procedure, using femoral vein cutdown, a catheter with an inflatable balloon at the tip is inserted and passed to the right atrium (Fig. 14–1). The operator then takes advantage of the fact that the foramen ovale of the interatrial septum remains "patent" at this stage of life. (The opening may be "functionally" closed by two membranes in apposition but yields to the tip of the catheter.) Thus, the catheter can be advanced across the septum into the left atrium. After confirmation of the location, the balloon is inflated with dilute contrast (3 to 3.5 ml, 1.6 to 2.0 cm diameter) and forcefully withdrawn into the right atrium, thereby creating a somewhat large functioning atrial

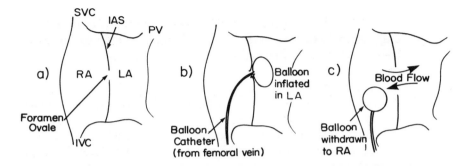

Fig. 14–1. Schematic representation of the Rashkind atrial septostomy procedure. A. Small opening in interatrial septum, through which a balloon catheter can be passed. B. Balloon inflated (about 2 cm in diameter) after passage into LA. C. Balloon forcefully withdrawn, rupturing an opening (about 2 cm^2) in the septum, which allows oxygenated blood to pass from the LA to the RA, and systemic venous blood (desaturated) to pass from the RA to the LA. (RA: right atrium. LA: left atrium. IVC: inferior vena cava. SVC: superior vena cava. IAS: interatrial septum. PV: pulmonary veins.)

septal defect. (It may be necessary to start with smaller volumes and repeat the process with larger volumes.) Significant amounts of blood can then interchange between the separate arterial and venous circulation, which raises systemic oxygenation considerably. Survival chances of the infant are improved with the opportunity to grow and attain a size that allows more definitive surgery to be undertaken.

The atrial septostomy technique is also applicable in infants with tricuspid atresia, total anomolous venous drainage, and other conditions in which creation of a large atrial septal defect with the balloon improves oxygenation.

Miscellaneous Techniques. Several other catheter "operations" have been developed for congenital heart disease. It is possible to insert devices by catheter techniques to close an atrial septal defect and a persistent ductus arteriosus. Such procedures are generally limited to laboratories specializing in congenital heart disease.

CATHETERIZATION FOR RETRIEVAL OF INTRAVASCULAR FOREIGN BODIES

On rare occasions, short lengths of plastic indwelling intravenous or central venous tubing inadvertently break off and are carried to right-heart chambers or the pulmonary artery. In the arterial circulation broken guidewire tips have become lodged in peripheral or even coronary arteries. The plastic tubing is radiopaque, so the fragment can usually be located by x ray. Wire tips are also seen on x ray.

Although not usually an acutely urgent complication, left in situ, these fragments may become a nidus of infection or thrombosis; they should therefore be removed. Ordinarily, this would entail thoracotomy or even open-heart surgery. However, a variety of snare devices using catheters have been developed that can obviate the need for major surgery. The particular snare used varies according to the exact location and length of the fragment. One fairly simple retrieval system will be described (Fig. 14–2). The components of the snare are a standard 100-cm, 8-French Lehman catheter and a 260- or 300-cm 0.18-in. Teflon-coated guidewire. Using sterile technique, both ends of the wire are inserted into the catheter tip so that they extend from the catheter hub. The two equal lengths of free wire are pulled until the wire loop at the catheter tip is about 1 cm in length. The apex of the loop is gently pulled into the tip of the catheter. The catheter is then inserted into the venous circulation by cutdown (arm vein) or percutaneously (femoral vein), depending on clinical circumstances and location of the fragment. The catheter tip is advanced until in the proximity of the fragment. One "limb" of the wire is pushed forward to form a soft flexible loop of wire that is variable in size. By catheter and loop manipulation the fragment can be trapped and snagged against the catheter tip by pulling back firmly on the wire. The catheter is then carefully withdrawn along with the trailing fragment.

A variation of this method uses a long suture tied to a flexible-tipped guidewire as a loop.

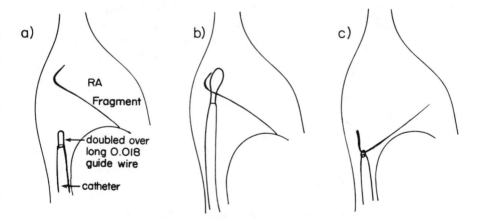

Fig. 14–2. *Schematic representation of snare removal of retained foreign body (e.g., a CVP catheter fragment). A. Radiopaque fragment lodged in the RA with end near tricuspid valve. The catheter is advanced from the femoral vein, with the enclosed snare, into the proximity of the fragment. B. The loop is advanced and hooked over the free end of the fragment. C. The snare is pulled down to snug the fragment against the tip of the catheter, and the catheter is withdrawn to extract the fragment.*

The removal of foreign bodies by this relatively simple, nonsurgical means always provides a sense of accomplishment for the laboratory personnel.

CARDIAC BIOPSY

The removal of small specimens of heart tissue can be useful in establishing certain cardiac diagnoses and following the progress of some conditions. In the past this required formal surgical thoracotomy or "blind" needle biopsy. However, more recently, a relatively simple and safe catheter technique has been developed for removal of small pieces from the right or left ventricular endomyocardium; it is known as endomyocardial biopsy (EMB). For example, EMB can establish the diagnosis of cardiac amyloidosis. The heart muscle is infiltrated and replaced by proteinaceous-like fibrils. The pathologist then examines the specimens microscopically after staining and by electron microscopy to make the diagnosis. Myocarditis and sarcoid of the heart are two other important conditions that can be detected with biopsy.

Considerable impetus for the development of modern biopsy technique has come from cardiac transplantation programs. Biopsies are frequently obtained to confirm the diagnosis of rejection and to observe the effects of immunosuppressive treatment. Finally, cancer therapeutic agents such as doxorubicin can have toxic effects on the heart and result in reduced cardiac function or overt congestive failure. Pathologic study of biopsy specimens from such hearts show histologic degeneration and a finding that would be reason to change or discontinue treatment. On the other hand, the absence of degenerative changes on biopsy can permit the use of larger and thus possibly more effective drug doses. Right ventricular EMB is more commonly performed and will be described. Left ventricular biopsy requires a somewhat different technique and can have a higher complication rate.

For RV biopsy (Fig. 14–3) the patient is prepared and monitored as for a standard right-heart catheterization. Informed consent is obtained. A bleeding diathesis, such as increased prothrombin time (greater than 15 or 16 sec.) or thrombocytopenia (less than 70,000 platelets) should not be present. The right neck area is draped. Standard percutaneous technique is used to insert a 9-French, 22- to 25-cm venous sheath into the jugular vein. The long sheath makes it possible for the tip to lie low in the superior vena cava, close to the right atrium. The standard biopsy device used in the United States and Great Britain is the Caves-Schultz bioptome, which is 50 cm long, 9 French, and semi-rigid, and has a handle that permits opening and closing of

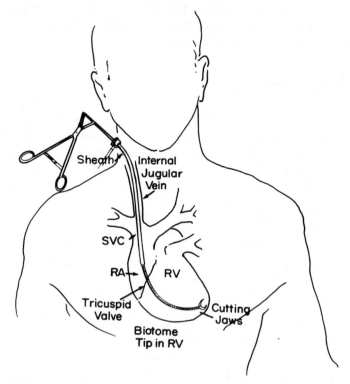

Fig. 14–3. Schematic representation of RV endomyocardial biopsy using the Caves-Schultz bioptome. The 9-French sheath has been inserted percutaneously into the right jugular vein, and the tip guided flouroscopically into the RA.

the cutting jaws at the tip. The operator inserts the tip (jaws closed) into the sheath, which guides the device safely through the venous channels into the larger cardiac chambers. Under fluoroscopy the tip is advanced across the tricuspid valve, into the right ventricle, and against the interventricular septum. The jaws are then opened, the device is pressed slightly against the septum, the jaws are firmly closed and, finally, the biopsy catheter is completely withdrawn. A few PVCs may occur as the jaws pull tissue away from the endomyocardium, but the patient generally has no unpleasant sensation. The jaws are then carefully examined under a strong light and the piece of tissue, about 2 mm^2, is picked out with a small needle (not forceps) and immediately placed in fixing solution. If possible a technician from the pathology department should be available to handle immediate fixation. A minimum of three specimens are taken for different types of processing.

The sheath is then removed and firm manual pressure is applied to the puncture site. The patient is assisted into the sitting position (which lowers venous pressure in the neck), and pressure is maintained for 10 min. An adhesive bandage is applied to the puncture site. Further observation of vital signs for ½ to 1 hour is usual after which, when appropriate, the patient can be accompanied home.

This procedure is associated with a low incidence of complications. Perforation into the pericardiac space can occur with hemopericardium, which might necessitate needle or surgical drainage. Injury to neck veins and bleeding at the puncture can also occur. Manipulation of the device from the right atrium to the right ventricle can cause arrhythmia.

BALLOON VALVULOPLASTY

The technology developed for transluminal balloon angioplasty, commonly applied in cases of stenotic lesion of the coronary and peripheral arteries, has been modified for dilating stenotic cardiac valves.

In adults the aortic valve becomes narrow, usually because of degenerative sclerosis and calcification and, less commonly now, because of rheumatic fever inflammation. When the stenotic aortic valve is less than 1.0 cm^2, the pumping function of the left ventricle decreases and clinical symptoms occur. An area of 0.5 cm^2 is critical. The main symptoms are syncope, angina, and congestive heart failure. Survival averages 2 to 3 years in patients with syncope or angina or both and less for patients with CHF.

Mitral valve stenosis is mainly a sequella of rheumatic fever endocarditis. Symptoms occur early in the course and may appear in patients in their late teens or twenties, particularly in less developed countries of the world. Fatigue, exercise intolerance, hemoptysis, arrhythmia (atrial fibrillation), and congestive failure are common. The stenotic valve is also prone to bacterial infection (endocarditis).

Since the development of cardiac surgery, particularly open-heart valve replacement, surgery has often been employed in the treatment of patients with aortic or mitral stenosis, with acceptable results. However, some patients with severe valvular stenosis are poor candidates for surgery (such as patients with concomitant severe pulmonary or renal insufficiency and aged patients). Such patients can be considered for the new technique of balloon valvuloplasty. A description of a procedure for aortic stenosis follows (Fig. 14–4).

Standard catheterization technique is used. Intra-arterial (radial or femoral) pressure monitoring is required in addition to the usual ECG. A right-heart thermal dilution catheter for pressure monitoring and cardiac output determination is in-

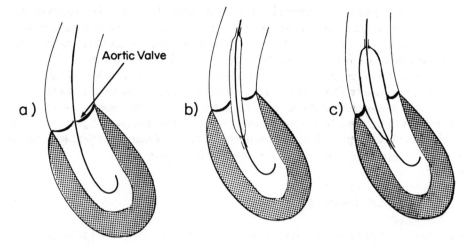

Fig. 14–4. Schematic representation of aortic balloon valvuloplasty. A. The J guidewire has been advanced across the stenotic aortic valve into the left ventricle. B. The balloon catheter is advanced over the guidewire and positioned in the aortic valve. C. The balloon is inflated, stretching and splitting the valve. The balloon is then deflated, resulting in an aortic valve with an increased area (preferably greater than 1.0 cm^2).

serted. The balloon valvuloplasty catheter has a large bore and is fairly stiff; the balloon length is 4 to 10 cm; inflated diameter is 10 to 20 mm. A 12-French sheath is inserted percutaneously into the right or left femoral artery. A standard pigtail or multipurpose catheter with a standard guidewire is advanced into the aortic root and then across the stenotic aortic valve into the left ventricle. (This can be a difficult maneuver). After withdrawing the guidewire and recording LV pressure, a long (300-cm) 0.038-in. guidewire with a large curve at the tip is reinserted into the catheter, and the tip is positioned in the left ventricle. The catheter is carefully withdrawn, retaining the tip of the long guidewire in the left ventricle. The valvuloplasty catheter can then be inserted over the long guidewire and positioned so the center of the balloon is at the aortic valve. The balloon is manually inflated with diluted contrast solution under fluoroscopy. The arterial pressure and ECG are monitored and the patient is observed. Inflation is maintained for 30 to 90 sec. if the patient reports no symptoms, the ECG is stable, and systolic pressure does not fall excessively (to less than 75 to 85 mmHg). The balloon is then deflated and the systolic gradient (pressure difference) between the LV and systemic artery is measured. Before valvuloplasty the gradient may be 100 mmHg or more; it should be significantly less after a successful dilation. Total elimination of the gradient is virtually impossible. A decrease to 20 mmHg would be acceptable. Several inflations may be required.

The mechanism of dilation includes fracture of calcific plates, commissural splitting, and stretching and displacement of rigid valve leaflets. "Normal" valve opening is not achieved, but the increase in area from 0.5 cm^2 to 1.0 cm^2 can result in dramatic clinical improvement. Complications include general vascular injury, laceration of the aortic ring (with resultant severe aortic regurgitation) and rarely calcific embolization. Restenosis occurs in at least 25% of patients.

This technique is now crude and transitional; future refinements are expected.

CATHETERS FOR ELECTRICAL STIMULATION OF THE HEART

Pacing Catheters. Electrode-tipped catheters have been in clinical use since 1959 for the treatment of rhythm disorders.

Patients with almost any form of heart disease can develop symptoms such as weakness, dizziness, or syncope because of an inadequate pulse rate (rhythm disorder), which may be acute or chronic. Sinus bradycardia or complete heart block may be the underlying mechanism. Sometimes complete heart block can result from acute myocardial infarction. When treatment is urgent, it is possible to insert a pacemaker wire (catheter) to provide temporary treatment until it is no longer necessary or until a permanent pacemaker can be implanted.

In many hospitals patients requiring temporary pacemakers are managed in a special procedure room of the cardiac care unit (with or without fluoroscopy) or in the ER; in hospitals without such units, the catheterization laboratory or x-ray department is commonly used.

The patient requires the usual preparation for a right-heart catheterization, although pressure, flow, and blood gas data are not generally obtained during such procedures.

Monitoring the ECG is vital. The pacing catheter or "wire" is generally solid (i.e., no lumen), constructed from woven Dacron or polyurethane, 80 to 125 cm long and 4 to 8 French (Fig. 6–6). It is fitted with two ring platinum electrodes close to the tip, 1.0 cm apart, with connecting pins or rings at the hub of catheter.

Pacing catheters are inserted by an arm vein cutdown or percutaneously through the subclavian or internal jugular vein. The femoral vein at the groin area can be used but is avoided because of the potential for infection with an indwelling catheter. The objective is to position the catheter tip with its bipolar electrodes in the apex of the right ventricle. When properly positioned, (under fluoroscopy) a sterile connecting cable is attached to the catheter electrodes; the other end is given to the assistant, who makes the connection to the pacemaker generator. The operator will direct the assistant to turn the generator on at a particular rate (e.g., 60 to 70 beats/min) and to slowly reduce the milliamps to determine pacing threshold, which should be less than 1 milliamp, indicating adequate electrode position. On the monitor a sharp pacing "spike" registers the same rate as that at which the pacemaker generator is set. Successful ventricular pacing is indicated by the spike, followed by a wide QRS complex occurring immediately after the spike (Fig. 14–5). Should pacing fail, for example, when the catheter tip is malpositioned or when stimulus strength is less than threshold, only the isolated spike appears. When pacing seems appropriate on the ECG monitor, the nurse or technician should feel the patient's pulse to be sure that the pulse is synchronous with ECG pacing.

The catheter is then fixed to the skin and a sterile dressing is applied, which also should be arranged to hold the wire firmly to avoid inadvertant withdrawal. It is vital that all electric connections be tight and insulated. Exposed electrode connections, if shorted, cause pacing to cease or, worse, conduct stray currents into the heart that could result in fatal fibrillation.

So-called "floating" pacing catheters are not ordinarily used in the catheterization laboratory, since fluoroscopy is available.

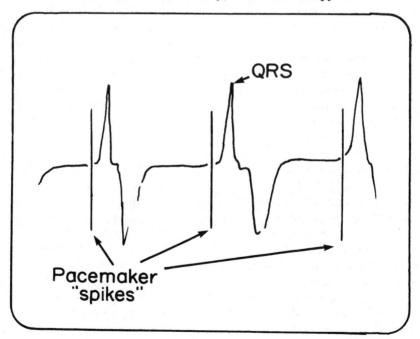

Fig. 14–5. Schematic representation of monitor screen with functioning pacemaker. The sharp "spikes" are the pacing artifact; the spikes induce a wide QRS complex from the ventricle.

Use of a pacing catheter for inducing arrhythmias for diagnostic and treatment purposes is discussed in chapter 3.

Catheter Tissue Ablation for Tachycardia. A relatively new and novel use for electrode catheters (similar to pacemaker catheters) is the delivery of electric currents to permanently prevent certain types of arrhythmia.

Tachyarrhythmia often originates in the atria or A-V junction and is conducted to the ventricles via the His bundle. In most clinical settings these cases of so-called supraventricular arrhythmia are not life-threatening or can be controlled with various antiarrhythmia drugs. In some patients, however, this kind of tachycardia can be almost incessant or may not respond to drugs, leading to clinical symptoms such as loss of consciousness and congestive heart failure. It is possible to surgically divide the His bundles and thus terminate the tachycardia. However, since this entails thoracotomy and open-heart surgery, the catheter technique can be substituted.

With a bipolar electrode catheter, the electrodes are positioned to record His bundle deflections, meaning that the electrodes are in close proximity to the His bundle itself. A direct electric current or radio frequency current is then passed through the electrodes, heating and injuring the bundle so it can no longer conduct impulses, thus terminating the tachycardia. Some injury to contiguous tissue may occur but should not be clinically significant. His bundle ablation requires subsequent permanent pacemaker implantation, because complete heart block is produced. This technique is not routine and can be considered experimental at this time.

SUMMARY

This chapter reviews several additional interventional catheterization techniques (see chapter 13 on vascular transluminal angioplasty). There is every reason to expect that the current procedures, which may seem crude, will be refined and that new, clever, catheter-facilitated procedures will be developed. Work is already in progress with lasers for angioplasty and fiberoptics for intravascular visualization.

15

General Operation and Equipment Inventory

Every catheterization laboratory has a specific way of managing "housekeeping" and record-keeping chores. Styles vary because of the interest and background of the director (who may be a radiologist, cardiologist, or pediatrician), the type of personnel working in the laboratory (nurse, x-ray technicians, or both), and the nature of the laboratory (research-oriented or service type). Following are practical suggestions for general operation that have been useful to me over the years and can serve as a study and orientation guide.

PRE-CATHETERIZATION CHECK LIST

Many details and tasks require attention in preparing the patient and the laboratory for a procedure. A checklist is therefore necessary to avoid oversights (Fig. 15–1). The list should be specifically tailored for each laboratory and retained in the patient's cath folder at the end of the procedure.

CATHETERIZATION PROCEDURE LOG

This is a basic worksheet or flowchart that is initiated when the patient arrives in the laboratory and undergoes preparation in the anteroom (Fig. 15–2). (A few of the items are redundant with the precatheterization checklist.) The worksheet is then used in the laboratory (on a clipboard) to record details of the conduct of the catheterization. The worksheet is completed at the end of the procedure and retained in the patient's cath folder.

CATH LAB LOGBOOK

The purpose of this logbook (Fig. 15–3) is to record, for statistical purposes, the details of each procedure as soon as it is completed.

CARDIAC CATHETERIZATION LABORATORY
PRE-CATH CHECK LIST

NAME_____ #_____DATE_____

_____ Call floor for Pre-Op.

_____ Called transport for patient

_____ Requested dentures from floor

_____ Patient arrived at_____

_____ Height and Weight

_____ Vitals signs taken

_____ Marked pulse (wrist or foot)

_____ Skin or pubic prep

_____ EKG discs placed

_____ Patient instruction given

_____ Mid-heart level marked

_____ Consent checked

_____ Lab test checked

_____ Allergies checked

_____ EKG on chart

_____ Lead 2 rhythm strip

_____ Ambu bag

_____ NTG Solution present

_____ Emergency drugs

_____ Crash cart checked

_____ Defibrillator on

_____ Anticipated materials ready

_____ Set-up tray

_____ Name tag on cine'

_____ Lab techs & intepreters notified

_____ Transducer level set

_____ Video tape

_____ Developer in recorder

_____ Recorder calibration

_____ Table positioned

_____ Table controls positioned

_____ Injector loaded

_____ Radiation badges worn

_____ Scouts taken

_____ ID card inserted

_____ Cut & cine' processor agitation

_____ Analytical machines on

_____ Requisitions stamped & prepared

_____ Patient data in log book

_____ H-P computer on

_____ Patient entered in computer

(Rev.4/89)

Fig. 15–1. Laboratory personnel use this checklist when preparing the patient and laboratory at the start of a procedure.

MOUNT SINAI HOSPITAL MEDICAL CENTER
CATHETERIZATION LAB REPORT

DATE 10/14/88   M.D. __SMITH__

PROCEDURE __LT/HEART/COR__ CASE # __350__

PAGE ☐
OF ☐   NAME AND HOSPITAL

     I D PLATE

PRE-PROCEDURE CHECK LIST

PT. ARRIVAL IN LAB __7:45__

I.D. VERIFICATION __YES__

CONSENT SIGNED __YES__

PRE-MEDICATION GIVEN __YES__

ALLERGIES __NONE__

ANTICOAGULANTS __NONE__

PRE-PROCEDURE INSTRUCTIONS __GIVEN__

HEIGHT __5'11''__ WEIGHT __172__

DENTURES __NONE__

PERTINENT MEDICAL HISTORY _____
     ANGINA - ON DILTIAZEM

EMERGENCY SUPPLIES/   YES
EQUIPMENT READY __YES__

LAB-DIAGNOSTIC RESULTS

PT __12/11.5__   PTT __22__

HGB __14.4__   HCT _____

BUN __18__   CREAT. __0.9__

K+ __4.1__   OTHER _____

ECG __IN CHART - N.S.R.__

CHEST X-RAY _____

OTHER _____

PRE-PROCEDURE VS · CARDIAC RHYTHM

BP __130/80__ PERIPHERAL PULSE-SITE ____

ASSESMENT __RIGHT DP/PT NORMAL__

MONITOR __ON__   6 LD. STRIP __DONE 76/MIN__

TIME __ PT. IN CATH. RM. __7:55 .__ _____ PROCEDURE BEGUN __8:05__

01	CUTDOWN/PUNCTURE INITIATED __LIDOCAINE RIGHT GROIN__
02	8 F ARTERIAL SHEATH - 8F PIGTAIL
03	HEPARIN 5000 U IA
05	AO AND LV PRESSURE - RANGE 100
08	LV ANGIO - 30° RAO 40 ML 10 ML/SEC - RENOGRAPHIN 76
09	LV PRESSURE -- AO RANGE 100
0:11	LEFT JUDKINS - 4 CM
0:17	LEFT COR ANGIOS - CHEST PAIN - IV NGL - RAPID RELIEF
0:24	LEFT COR ANGIO X 5
0:26	RIGHT JUDKINS - RT COR ANGIOS X 3
0:32	CATH OUT - PROTAMINE IV 40 MG
0:37	SHEATH OUT
0:47	NO BLEEDING - PRESSURE DRESSING - FOOT PULSES NORMAL - COLOR GOOD

_____ CLOSURE BEGUN _____

_____ CLOSURE COMPLETE _____ DRESSING (TYPE/SITE) _____
_____ SITE ASSESSMENT _____
__8:55__ POST PROCEDURE BP __125/80__ HR __85__ MONITOR _____
_____ POST PROCEDURE INSTRUCTIONS __GIVEN__ DISCHARGE FROM LAB ____

MIDHEART __60__ IT DISTANCE __96__ SCREEN __30__ FRAMES __30__ CONTRAST MEDIUM __95 ML__

Fig. 15–2. *Catheterization procedure log. Entries (shown here in type for clarity) are made by hand during the course of a procedure. A continuation sheet (not shown) is often needed.*

It takes only a few moments to enter the data when they are fresh in one's mind. The columns can be added at the bottom as each page is completed; periodic totals are tabulated at appropriate intervals (monthly, semi-annually, annually, etc.). The physician will usually enter the data, but a nurse or technician can easily do it also.

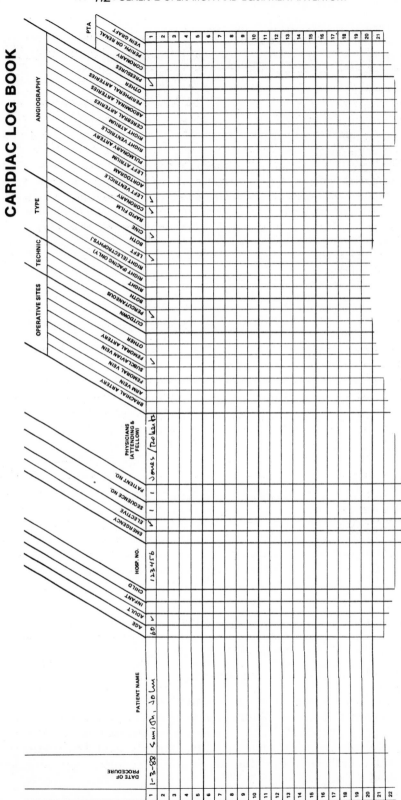

Figure 15-3. *First half of cardiac log book. See full legend below second half on facing page.*

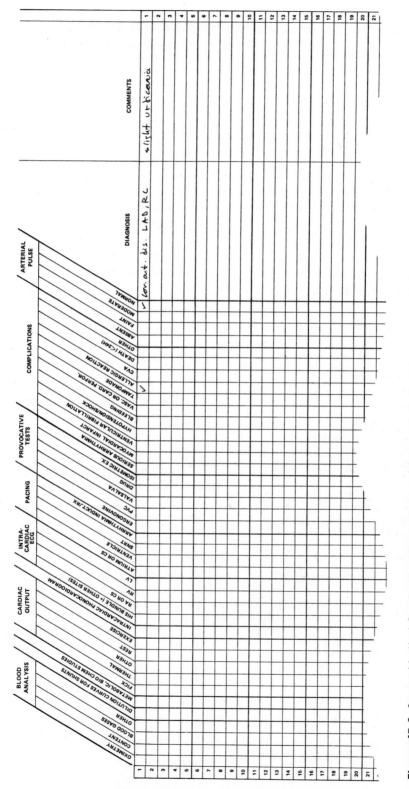

Figure 15-3. Second half of Cardiac Log Book. These pages are actually 11 in. × 16 in. and are held in a large looseleaf binder, which is kept in a conspicuous place in the laboratory. Entries should be made as soon as a procedure is completed.

This system might be considered antiquated and could easily be replaced by a computerized data-acquisition system. The manual system, however, has the advantage of simplicity, and the log is always available for immediate review.

INSTRUMENT TRAY—PACKS

The following tray setups are to be considered models that can and should be modified to suit the needs of each laboratory. For efficiency's sake, agreement should be reached by those working in a laboratory to design a "percutaneous tray" and a "cutdown tray." The total number of trays needed will depend on the caseload of the laboratory and the preparation "turnaround" time. Table 15–1 outlines a sample percutaneous tray, and Table 15–2 outlines a sample cutdown tray.

Table 15–1. *Percutaneous Tray (Packed and Sterilized).*

2 Sponge bowls
1 Beaker, 125 ml (for betadine)
1 Doz. gauze 4 × 4
2 Large towel clamps
2 Large curved clamps
2 Small curved clamps
1 Large sponge clamp
1 Scalpel-blade holder
1 No. 11 scalpel blade
2 Medicine cups (for lidocaine, heparin)
1 "Control" syringe, 10 ml (can be omitted if disposable is used)

Add the following disposable items after tray is opened on surgical table or cart:
1 Large aperture drape (disposable)
1 25-gauge ½-in. needle
1 20-gauge ½- – 2-in. needle
1 18-gauge Seldinger-type needle
3 Plastic syringes, 10 ml
1 Plastic syringe, 5 ml

Heparin solution (2500 IU/500 ml 5% D/W) to half fill sponge bowls.
8 ml each of 2% lidocaine and heparin (1000 IU/ml) in each medicine cup (place lidocaine cup at left-upper part of setup, heparin cup at right-lower part, or use some other scheme that *never* varies)*
I.V. tubing for dye and solutions
Pressure-line tubing (to strain gauge)
Pressure-line tubing for injector
Morse 3 stop-cock manifold**

Sheaths, guidewires, puncture needle, and catheters will be requested by the physician-operator, depending on the procedure.

*An additional precaution is to place a small piece of colored tape on the lidocaine cup and syringe.
**For ease of use, we have requested the supplier to modify the manifold so the flag handles point to "closed" (see Fig. 9–1).

The cutdown tray requires more instruments than the percutaneous tray. Cutdown trays can be used for both venous and arterial procedures.

At the completion of a procedure the nurse or technician (wearing rubber gloves) discards all non-reusable material in a large container to be considered contaminated. Reusable instruments are collected, carefully washed and dried, and reassembled in the appropriate traypack. Bent or rusting instruments should be discarded. Cleaning of instruments and assembling trays should be done in a clean utility room.

Table 15–2. Cutdown Tray.

2 Large towel clamps	2 Small curved hemostats
2 Small towel clamps	1 Medium curved hemostat
1 Iris forceps (straight)	1 Large curved hemostat
1 Iris forceps (curved)	1 Medium right-angle clamp
1 Large surgical scissor	1 Pair small Army/Navy retractor
1 Fine surgical scissor	2 Scalpel-blade holders
1 Large needle holder (skin)	1 No.-11 scalpel blade
1 Fine needle holder (artery)	1 No.-15 scalpel blade
4 Small straight hemostats	1 Large sponge clamp
1 Fine-toothed tweezers	2 Sponge bowls
1 Mouse-toothed tweezers	2 Medicine cups (lidocaine, heparin)
1 Beaker, 125 ml (betadine)	6-0 Braided polyester suture (arterial needle)
1 Control syringe, 10 ml*	3-0 Silk or polyester suture (skin needle)
1 Doz. gauze 4 × 4	Disposables**

*Omit if disposable used.
**Add the disposables, as listed in Table 15-1, after the sterile traypack is opened on the surgical table or cart. Heparin 5000 IV/1000 ml is added to all flush solutions.

GENERAL CATHETERIZATION LABORATORY EQUIPMENT

Defibrillator: Nurses and physicians, and possibly other technicians, should be able to operate the defibrillator. It is turned on and tested every day, and checked monthly by the hospital bioengineering service.

Suction machine: This can be portable or wall-operated; it is used in case of vomiting and after intubation.

Oxygen supply

Intubation equipment (laryngoscopes, endotracheal tubes): It is helpful if a member of the team has experience in intubation, but the equipment should be available for the on-call anesthesiologist.

Ambu-bag

Automatic BP cuff: This is useful when one nurse is assisting in resuscitation. All equipment requires periodic testing and servicing.

Automated I.V. drip controls (IVACS)

CATHETERIZATION EQUIPMENT: INVENTORY AND STORAGE

Aside from the general surgical instruments, the specific equipment for catheterization includes cardiac catheters, introducer sheaths, guidewires, and puncture needles. Angiographic dye is the main pharmacologic diagnostic agent. All of these items are available from several different companies; there are small but important differences between typical generic items. The laboratory director will generally indicate the variety of catheters and other instruments that should be stocked, and from which vendors they should be purchased. Some laboratories function in a consortium with others to obtain bulk discounts.

Stock will vary, depending on whether the laboratory functions primarily for cardiology, radiology, pediatrics, or combinations thereof. For example, most radiology laboratories use percutaneous equipment almost exclusively, and will thus have essentially no use for catheters inserted by cutdown (such as the Sones catheter).

A wide range of catheter shapes, sizes, and lengths are needed to meet the variety of procedure goals and differing patient requirements. The inventory size will depend on the caseload, the efficiency of the purchasing mechanism, and how long it takes to receive requisitioned items.

The same considerations exist for sheaths, wires, and other instruments, all of which are available in wide varieties for different purposes.

In laboratories that perform peripheral and coronary angiography the problem is more complex, again because of the vast array of balloon catheters, steering wires, special introducers, and other instruments. Coronary balloon catheters are priced in excess of $600 each (1989).

An accurate inventory must be kept so purchasing can be initiated on a timely basis. In our laboratory we use a simple system. Each category of equipment has a corresponding inventory sheet (Fig. 15–4). The main features of this sheet are: nominal supply stock, number of items in stock, and reorder number (i.e., the number of a given item in stock at which the item is reordered). These numbers depend on the laboratory utilization rate and how long it takes an item to reach the laboratory after reordering (experience shows this is always longer than expected). The laboratory obviously maintains a larger stock of commonly used items and reorders these more frequently.

Each day the nurse or technician keeps a tally of all items used for each procedure. For example, at the end of a day the equipment used might include:

JUDKINS - LEFT CORONARY

SIZE	LENGTH	CAT#		NOMINAL	REORDER
8F-3.5	100	523-838	23, 21	25	12
8F-4	100	523-840	45, 43, 42, 40	50	25
8F-5	100	523-842	35, 34	40	20
8F-6	100	523-844	45, 24	30	15
7F-3.5	100	523-718	9, 8	10	5
7F-4	100	523-720	18, 16, 15	20	10
7F-5	100	523-722	8, 7	10	5
7F-6	100	523-724	4, 3	5	3

Fig. 15–4. *Typical inventory sheet. "Nominal" is the full laboratory stock. Purchasing is initiated when the inventory level falls to "Reorder." The numbers chosen are arbitrary and will vary from lab to lab. The handwritten numeric entries show catheter utilization. For example, under 8F-4, initial catheter inventory was 45, but on three occasions 2, then 1, then 2 catheters were used, leaving a current inventory of 40.*

2 8-French Judkins pigtails
2 8-French Judkins left (4-cm) and right (4-cm) coronary catheter
1 7-French Judkins pigtail
1 7-French left (4-cm) and 1 7-French right (4-cm) coronary catheter
1 8-French Eppendorf (100 cm)
2 8-French arterial sheaths
2 7-French arterial sheaths
4 0.035-in. J guidewires
1 0.035-in. straight guidewire
3 18-gauge arterial puncture needles

The nurse or technician now records this information on the appropriate inventory sheet (all maintained in order in a loose-leaf binder). For example if two 8-French, 4-cm pigtails are used, and the last entry shows 20 remaining, the "20" is crossed out and replaced by "18." Thus, the inventory is constantly up-to-date, obviating the need for periodic complete inventory-taking by hand (which is very time-consuming).

This system, although easy to use once in place, will easily adapt to computerization, which may be more efficient in large, busy laboratories (with multiple catheterization suites).

GENERAL CATHETERIZATION EQUIPMENT INVENTORY

Literally hundreds of catheters and other devices are available from at least three major manufacturers. Some of these devices are frequently used, others rarely, but each laboratory requires an extensive inventory to be ready to perform both the usual and unusual procedure.

Tables 15–3, 15–4, and 15–5, which list and describe catheters, guidewires, and sheaths, respectively, can be considered reasonably representative and would be modified depending on the specific needs of the laboratory. Angioplasty equipment is not included because requirements are very specific and the technology is in considerable flux. Transeptal puncture technique equipment is also not included.

Table 15–3. Catheters.*

Type	Use
Judkins left coronary (femoral) 7 and 8 French, 3.5–6 cm curve**	Standard percutaneous transfemoral coronary angiography
Judkins right coronary (femoral) 7 and 8 French, 3.5–6 cm curve	Standard percutaneous transfemoral coronary angiography
Pigtail 6–8 French, 100 cm; 5–8 French, 65 cm	Standard percutaneous transfemoral ventriculography or aortography
Femoral renal 7 and 8 French	Percutaneous renal angiography
Femoral multipurpose 7 and 8 French	Percutaneous transfermoral, ventriculography, aortography
Femoral coronary vein bypass, right and left	Aorto-coronary vein graft angiography
Femoral internal mammary 7 and 8 French	Internal mammary angiography
Femoral cerebral (head-hunter) 7 and 8 French (normal modified dilated arch, dilated arch)	Cerebral angiography (commonly used by radiologists)
Sones coronary woven Dacron 7 and 8 French, standard tip (1.5 cm) and short tip (1.0 cm)	Standard transbrachial coronary angiography; can also be used for ventriculography
Eppendorf (woven Dacron) 6–8 French	Right-heart angiography, pulmonary LV angiography and aortography
Pediatric NIH (woven Dacron) 4–6 French	Pediatric angiography
Lehman woven Dacron 5–8 French	Right-heart pressures
Goodale-Lubin woven Dacron 5–8 French	Right-heart pressures
Swan-Ganz polyethylene 7.5 French, 4 lumen, (thermal)	Right-heart pressures; cardiac output

*Unless indicated catheters are made from polyurethane. The percutaneous catheters are also available in polyethylene.
**5-French high-flow catheters are now available for coronary angiography.

Table 15–4. Guidewires.

Property	Type	Comment
Coating	All Teflon	Smooth passage, reduced thrombogenicity
Core	Fixed	Standard flexible end
	Movable	Allows adjustment in length of flexible end segment
Tip configuration	Straight	Standard
	3-mm J or 6-mm J	For negotiating tortuous vessels
Length	145–150 cm	Standard
	280–300 cm	"Exchange" wire
Diameter	0.018 in.	For very-small-bore or Swan-Ganz catheters
	0.035–0.038 in.	Standard

Table 15–5. Sheaths.*

Size	Use
5–8 French (length is 11 cm for adult, 9 cm for pediatric)	Standard catheter insertion; the 7- or 7.5-French Swan catheter requires an 8-French sheath
9 French (length is 25–40 cm)	Used for RV bioptome

*Usually fitted with a hemostasis valve and side-arm.

MISCELLANEOUS EQUIPMENT

Puncture Needles. Most operators use an 18-gauge thin-wall needle cannula for femoral artery and vein punctures. For jugular vein puncture, needle/sheaths can be used and are supplied in the usual commercially available kits.

IV Tubing. A variety of tubing is used to connect flush and dye reservoir to the manifold. Pressure-resistant tubing connects catheters to power injectors

Drapes. Disposable paper drapes have replaced material toweling and sheets. Drapes are available with small exposure holes for femoral or arm procedures.

CHARGE ACCOUNTING

Each laboratory has a system, worked out in conjunction with the hospital business administration, to submit charge slips after completing a procedure. There may be 20 to 25 different procedure descriptions used, which could be in code form. The breakdown usually begins with "right-" or "left-" heart catheterization (or is combined), and is modified by the type of angiography and other factors.

16

Quality Control and Assurance

Quality control and assurance (QC and QA) concepts, borrowed from engineering, have recently been applied to certain aspects of medicine. Reputable catheterization laboratories kept track of and assessed the results of their procedures long before they came under the scrutiny of government and accreditation agencies. Currently, there are specific requirements for laboratories to collect and analyze data and take corrective action if necessary. However, since there is no definitive format to accomplish this, QA practices vary from laboratory to laboratory. The following discussion of QC and QA measures is not intended to be complete or exhaustive. Some of these measures are undoubtedly practiced in almost all laboratories; it is important for nursing and technician personnel to have a basic understanding of the principles.

RADIATION SAFETY

(General procedure is discussed in chapter 8).

All x-ray equipment requires periodic testing to make sure that there is proper x-ray dosing to the patient and that scatter controls are functioning. The data are obtained by a radiation physicist and reported to the appropriate state agency (the specific responsible department varies from state to state).

Film badge data are collected and reviewed by the hospital radiation safety officer (or committee) and the laboratory director. If individual badges show radiation exposure beyond recommended limits, an attempt is made to help the individual reduce exposure by such measures as spending less time in the x-ray room, maximizing distance from the x-ray source, and improving shielding. Exceeding the "limit" on a badge is a warning and does not by itself imply a particular health hazard.

FILM PROCESSING QUALITY

A standard technique of testing the processing quality of cine film is to expose a test strip with a controlled light sensitometer,

120

process the film in the usual way, and examine the strip with a densitometer. The results of the tests are recorded so that deviations are apparent and corrective measures can be taken.

INFECTION CONTROL

This issue was briefly mentioned in chapter 5. Maintaining cleanliness of the laboratory and maintaining equipment sterility are important tasks for nursing and technician personnel.

Any unusual infection or increased incidence is reported to the infection control officer or committee for analysis of the problem and recommendations. As noted, infection in modern laboratories is rare.

All disposable items coming into contact with the patient are considered to be contaminated and are deposited in designated receptacles. (Sheeting is now essentially all disposable.) To some degree this is a response to the current problem of AIDS.

AIDS is also the reason for the current requirement that goggles must be worn by an individual close enough to be spattered by blood, e.g., in the case of a brachial artery cutdown procedure.

In some hospitals, the laboratory and equipment are bacteriologically tested periodically for inappropriate contaminants. The results are reported to the infection control officer (or committee) for remedial action if needed.

The hospital infection control committee and laboratory director usually develop written infection control protocols, which are periodically reviewed and updated.

PROCEDURE COMPLICATIONS

A laboratory log (see Fig. 15–3) should be maintained to make it relatively easy for a nurse or lab technician to periodically collate complication data. This is done annually in our laboratory, and the data are distributed to the attending cardiologists for information and comment. When a particular complication occurs beyond a reasonable standard (determined by the director), corrective action is required.

Some laboratories have a formal mechanism whereby the laboratory director or a committee of cardiologists will review fatalities in the laboratory (usually defined as death occurring in the laboratory or within 24 hours of the procedure, later if the death is a direct result of an incident in the laboratory). Review does not necessarily imply inappropriate performance or procedure and should be viewed as an educational effort. Nursing and technician personnel may be asked for their observations and comments. Records will be maintained of such proceedings to demonstrate awareness of the problem and to recognize trends. These records should be treated as confidential documents. Corrective action may follow.

Following a cardiac arrest (usually ventricular fibrillation) during a procedure, laboratory personnel should fill out an arrest protocol log for review with the director. Items of concern include: promptness of recognition of the event, promptness in instituting resuscitation measures, personnel knowing their responsibilities, and proper function of equipment (defibrillator, laryngoscope, suction, etc.). Corrective action is undertaken in areas found inadequate.

CONFERENCES

Some form of continuing education is an important element of QA. This can have many formats, including didactic lectures, reviewing educational audio or video tapes (which unfortunately are geared mainly to the physician but still may be useful for other personnel), and case presentations. In larger laboratories the laboratory supervisor can organize much of the program.

In our laboratory we find it possible to hold a weekly conference in which nearly all cases from the previous week are presented. In addition to the nursing and technical staff, the cardiology fellows, residents and students, and the attending physician involved with procedure are expected to attend the conference. Although the medical aspects of the case are emphasized (patient history, indications for the procedures, findings, clinical correlation, and recommendations), the nonphysician personnel have an opportunity to become familiar with general medical issues and controversies pertaining to catheterization, rather than concentrating only on technical aspects. Although hard to demonstrate with statistics, such involvement should lead to improved performance. Records of the procedures are maintained, which are available for QA analysis.

SUMMARY

This chapter outlines some of the ways that laboratory activities are monitored to maintain technical quality and safety for patients and personnel. Topics include radiation, infection, complications, and education.

Appendix

PROCEDURE CHARGE ACCOUNTING AND RELATIVE VALUE SYSTEM

It is important for catheterization laboratories and radiology special procedure units and hospitals to use a simple, realistic, and easily adjusted procedure charge system. Our system consists of unit blocks with add-ons that depend on procedure complexity. As an example, we can consider a right-heart catheterization as a basic unit. If a pulmonary angiogram is also obtained, this is an additional procedure unit and generates an add-on charge. The table is thus constructed, for the most part, by starting with basic procedures such as right-heart catheterization, left-heart catheterization, right- and left-heart catheterization, and aortography, and expands through the addition of procedure elements. The list encompasses the majority of diagnostic and therapeutic procedures. (Balloon valvuloplasty and laser angioplasty are not included.)

Since the procedure list is based on a building-block system, it is possible to assign relative values to procedures of different complexities (right column). Once the relative values are in place, the unit value can be given a hospital- and laboratory-specific value by the hospital finance department.

The relative value system shown here is not designed to include the physician-input component. (It might be appropriate to include such a component when a hospital directly employs physicians to do the procedures. A separate system might also be devised for physicians compensated by fee-for-service.)

The following factors have been considered in developing the relative values: nurse and technician time and input intensity, procedure time, use of fixed catheterization laboratory equipment, and use of consumables such as film, dye, pharmacologicals and, nowadays, very expensive items such as angioplasty equipment. The weighting is clearly somewhat arbitrary and should be adjusted for the particular circumstances of the laboratory.

Some of the basic relative value blocks that have been included in the system are:

Right-heart catheterization:	100
First angiogram:	40
Additional angiogram:	20
Coronary angiograms:	50

PTCA adds 150 units to a basic right- and left-heart procedure with coronary angiograms because of the costly additional equipment and procedure time.

This system, unlike some in use elsewhere, does not require the laboratory personnel to add points based on the exact length of procedure time, how many diagnostic catheters are used, length of cine film, and other considerations. Enough procedures are performed in most laboratories for a procedure-specific relative value to represent an average.

The cost accountant utilizes somewhat different methods at arriving at cost and charges. However, in analyzing data at Mount Sinai Hospital in Chicago and scaling the dollar cost of the relative value unit, there is a rather close correspondence between the two methods. The scaling of the unit value should be made hospital-specific. As costs (inevitably) rise, it is a simple matter, when necessary, to adjust the unit relative value and avoid the need to make changes in individual procedure charges.

Procedure List.

Procedure	Units
Right-heart cath	100
Right-heart cath + 1 angio	140
Right-heart cath + 2 angios	160
Right-heart cath + 3 angios	180
Right-heart cath + 4 angios	200
Venous angio (any site: e.g., IVC)	140
Electrophysiologic study, complete	200
Right atrial pacing/HB study only	100
Cardiac output or diagnostic run (oxygen saturation) add	25
Left-heart cath	125
Right- & left-heart cath	150
Left-heart cath + 1 angio	165
Left-heart cath + 2 angios	185
Left-heart cath + 3 angios	205
Left-heart cath + 1 angio + coronaries	225
Left-heart cath + 2 angios + coronaries	245
Left-heart cath + 3 angios + coronaries	265
Right- & left-heart cath + 1 angio	190
Right- & left-heart cath + 2 angios	210
Right- & left-heart cath + 3 angios	230
Right- and left-heart cath + 1 angio + coronaries	250

Right- and left-heart cath + 2 angios + coronaries..............270
Right- and left-heart cath + 3 angios + coronaries..............290

Aortogram—any site..160
Aortogram—2nd injection add...................................... 40
Aortogram + 1 sel. arteriogram (e.g., arch study + 1
   cereb. vessel...180
Aortogram + 2 sel. arteriograms (e.g., abd. flush
   & bilat. renals)..200
Aortogram + 3 sel. arteriograms 220
Aortogram + 4 sel. arteriograms 240

Selective arteriogram (sep. proc) 1 vessel.....................150
Selective arteriogram   2 vessels 170
Selective arteriogram   3 vessels 190
Selective arteriogram   4 vessels 210
Selective arteriogram   5 vessels 230

PTA—1 entry...225
PTA—2 entries 275

Atherectomy—1 entry...300
Atherectomy—2 entries 350
Atherectomy—2nd instrument add...................................... 50

Femoral or brachial arteriogram—1 entry...........................125
Femoral or brachial arteriogram—2 entries 150

PTCA—1 vessel 400
PTCA—2 vessels...450
PTCA—3 vessels..500

Cath Lab Procedures: Miscellaneous.

Procedure	Units
Cancel/incomplete study	25
Fluoroscopy	25
Plain cine	40
Temporary pacemaker	100
Permanent pacemaker	150
Foreign-body retrieval	150
Pericardiocentesis	150
Cardioversion	50
Endocardial biopsy (R or L)	175
Biplane any angio add	20

Index

Page numbers in italics indicate figures; those followed by "t" indicate tables; those followed by "n" indicate footnotes.

A

AIDS, 121
Air purging, of injectors, 71
Alcohol, heart damage by, 58
Allergic reactions
  diabetic patients and, 80
  management of, 80
  to contrast media, 67-69
  to protamine, 80
Amyloid, cardiac granuloma, 11
Anesthesia, local, 25, 39-40, 42
Angiography
  complications of, 73-76
  contrast media used in, 67, 69, 71
  myocardial infarction during, 29
  of aorta, 70, 72-73
  of coronary arteries, 3, 73-76
  of left ventricle, 72, 74
  of peripheral vessels, 14, 70
  of pulmonary arteries, 68n, 72
  pediatric, 72
Angioplasty. See also Valvuloplasty
  atherectomy catheter and, 96
  complications of, 89
  drill mediated, 95-96
  experimental techniques in, 95-96
  history of, 85-86
  in coronary arteries, 89-95, 90
  in peripheral vessels, 86-88, 88
  in vein grafts, 94
  laser mediated, 95
  restenosis after, 88, 93
Antiarrhythmic drugs, 81-82
Anticoagulants, 79-80, 90
Antihistamines, 69
Aorta
  angiography of, 70, 72-73
  coarctation of, 12-13
  congenital heart disease and, 12
  normal pressure in, 57t
  oxygen saturation and, 65t
  visceral branches of, 14
Aortic valve
  area of, 61, 62
  regurgitation, 14
  stenosis of, 104-106, 105

Aortic valvular insufficiency, 73
Arrhythmia
  contrast media and, 27-28, 69, 75-76
  His bundle and, 15, 108
  medication for, 15, 78, 80-82
Arterial insufficiency, 14, 42
Arteries. See names of individual arteries
Arteriovenous oxygen difference, 61
Aspirin, 79, 86
Atherectomy catheters, 96
Atheromatous plaque. See Atherosclerotic plaque
Atherosclerotic plaque, 14
  experimental removal of, 95-96
  in coronary arteries, 89-95, 90
  in peripheral arteries, 86-88, 88
  interference with catheter, 48
Atrial septal defect, 64, 99-100, 100
Atrial septum
  catheterization through, 46
  congenital defect in, 64, 100
  septostomy of, 99-100, 100
Atropine, 80-81
Automatic intracardiac defibrillator, 27

B

Bacterial endocarditis, and drug abuse, 10
Balloon catheters, 3, 35-36, 37
  in angioplasty, 87-94, 88, 90, 94
  in atrial septostomy, 99-100, 100
  in valvuloplasty, 104-106, 105
  thrombi removal with, 41
Beta blockers, 81
Biopsy, cardiac, 102-104, 103
"Birds-eye" catheter, 32
Birth defects. See Congenital heart disease
Bleeding
  as complication, 29, 73, 98
  at catheter insertion site, 41, 44, 45, 48
  cutdowns and, 40-41
Blood clots. See Thrombi
Blood flow system, 63, 65